The TAO of NAD

Unlock the Secrets to Vitality and Longevity: Supercharge Your Cells and Spirit with NAD and Ancient Taoist Wisdom

By JIn-XIONG SHE, PhD

FOUNDER, CEO AND CHIEF SCIENTIFIC OFFICER OF JINFINITI PRECISION MEDICINE

Edited by Kevin Rush

Cover Design by Doni Waikel, coversbydoni.com

Book Cover Photograph of Author by Peggy McIntaggart Seagren

ISBN: 978-1-965971-16-1

DEDICATION

To my father, Keshu She — the man who instilled in me an unshakable discipline and relentless drive. His example taught me that hard work and perseverance are the backbone of success.

To my mother, Yuanfeng Zhu — who gave me the most powerful gift of all: self-confidence. She made sure that every time I stepped out into the world, I carried with me the unwavering belief that I had what it takes to achieve whatever I set my mind to.

This little Chinese guy owes an immeasurable debt of gratitude to two extraordinary people from Songzhi, who instilled in their children a profound truth: it is not nationality, color, race, gender, or perceived limitations that define us. Character is what matters. And for that, I am forever grateful.

ACKNOWLEDGMENTS

This book is the distillation of my more than four decades of study, research, and experimentation. More than that, it is informed by observations derived from the literature on the health outcomes of tens of thousands of patients of physicians from all parts of the world. When you factor in the thousands of people who have consulted with me as the founder of my own wellness company and my own life experiences of more than 60 years, you begin to get a sense of the scope of what I've learned. Add my personal philosophical overlay, and you are holding in your hand a unique, hybrid guide to extending healthspan.

Books don't come to life in a vacuum, and this one is no exception. I owe thanks to people, places, and things. First, I want to voice my appreciation to the thousands of students who learned under my tutelage in classes ranging from Genetics to Precision Medicine. It was their eager and inspiring quest for knowledge and hard science facts that fueled countless early morning classes I taught and long hours preparing salient coursework.

Next, without the support of friends and colleagues, the decision to transition from academia to the business world would have been nearly impossible. There is a lot of agreement in the world that attaining a tenured position as a professor, having a 30,000-square-foot building built in your honor over which you have dominion, and publishing over 400 papers are the foundation for a cushy state of semi-retirement. To those who understood my passion to make a difference now in the lives of people everywhere, I say, "Thank you!" To those who have helped me create *Jinfiniti* Precision Medicine, I salute you for the long hours and endless days that it takes to build something from scratch.

Haitao Liu, I appreciate you not just because you are my nephew, but because you are steadfast and unwavering in your ability to work long hours and put in the deep thinking and mental diligence that are your signature traits.

Bob Thordarson, you have been with me since the beginning, offering your business insights and objective opinions. We don't always agree, but we never spend a moment on anything less than material matters. Greta Blackburn, you drove me crazy pushing me to write this book and helping to make it happen. Without your hard work and motivation, it might have languished as "an idea" for who knows how long?

Kevin Rush, your talent as a writer informed the suggestions and edits you contributed and without them, this book would not have the same feel or flow. To my colleagues and peers in the longevity field, thank you for sharing a vision of what the New 100 looks like.

There are so many doctors with whom I share friendship and a passion for this great movement of which we are all members.

Last but not least, I could not do what I do without the support and love of my family. My wife, Dr. Boying Dun, is a brilliant scientist in her own right. She is a tireless partner who inspires me daily. On top of that she is a loving mother to our two daughters, Lily and Jasmine. They are the light and loves of my life. Balance is one of my 8 Pillars of TAO, and my family, along with my beloved game of tennis are what keep me balanced and allow me to be the best I can be.

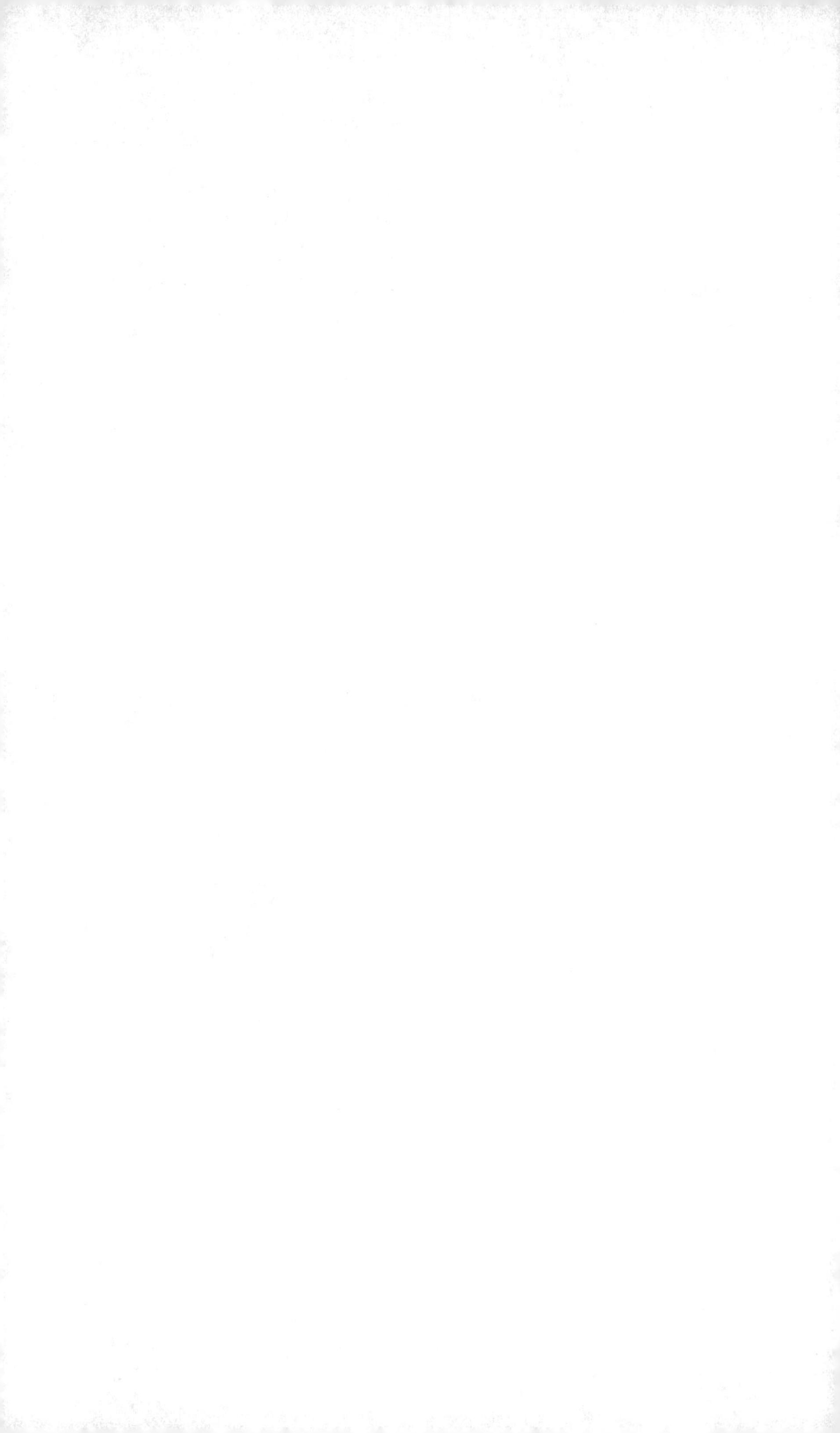

TABLE OF CONTENTS

FOREWORD

In an era where modern medicine continuously advances yet struggles to address chronic disease and longevity holistically, Dr. Jin-Xiong She offers a refreshing, integrative perspective—one that bridges the ancient wisdom of TAO with the rigor of Western science. This book is more than just a guide; it is a revelation, demonstrating how timeless Eastern principles, when paired with cutting-edge research, can lead to better health outcomes, greater vitality, and a longer, healthier life.

The global chorus of testimonials from doctors, scientists, and wellness experts underscores the significance of Dr. She's work. His approach speaks to a growing realization: that true health and longevity cannot be achieved by focusing on just one philosophy, one system, or one discipline alone. The most effective solutions today arise from an amalgamation of what has been scientifically validated across different traditions. The TAO framework he presents acts as a unifying force, seamlessly weaving together the best aspects of eastern wisdom and Western Medicine.

At first glance, some of the principles laid out in this book may appear simple. But therein lies their power. Simplicity, when rooted in logic and backed by science, often holds the deepest truths. Dr. She has mastered the art of distilling complex biological and philosophical insights into actionable strategies—proving that in health, as in nature, less is often more.

With this book, you are invited to step into a new paradigm of health—one that does not reject modern medicine but enhances it with the harmony and balance of TAO. It is a long-overdue perspective, and one that, if embraced, has the potential to redefine how we approach well-being in the 21st century.

Let this book be your guide.

Greta Blackburn
Founding Editor, Ms. Fitness Magazine
Developer and Co-Author of The Immortality Edge, *the world's first prescriptive book on Telomere Biology*

TESTIMONIALS

"The world of anti-aging medicine is a cornucopia of cultures, disciplines, practices, and protocols. Dr. She brings the wisdom of the Chinese tradition of TAO to the mix. In this book he makes a compelling case for NAD optimization and biomarker testing as a powerful and organic extension of TAO philosophy."

Luis Martinez, MD
Founder, Caribbean Anti-Aging Medicine Association (CAAMAS)and Xanogene Clinics
Co-Founder, Clinical Peptide Society
Co-Founder, Senolytic Therapy Network

"The Age Management Medicine Group is founded upon the belief that health and wellness professionals should provide collaborative, holistic, and science-based care. We educate in total wellness: nutrition, exercise, proper supplementation, informed diagnostics, and continuing education.

Dr. She has delivered a book that informs people about the powerful and proven principles of TAO. These, combined with his extensive science, research, and data background, create a useful guide that can provide effective fundamentals for managing age-related decline."

Rick Merner
Co-Founder, Age Management Medicine Group (AMMG)

"My journey into biohacking began under the guidance of Dr. She. As a performer, I need the most energy, creativity, and mental focus I can muster for extended worldwide tours and packed conferences. When you work with the Fortune 100 and the likes of Santana, Madonna, Earth, Wind and Fire and the teams behind Lady GaGa and Bruno Mars, you have to bring your "A" game every time. This book and the powerful diagnostic tools and supplements created under the guidance of Dr. She at his company, Jinfiniti Precision Medicine, help me to do just that!"

Freddie Ravel
International Transformational Keynote Speaker, Life in Tune® Founder, Grammy-Nominated Artist, and Biohacker

---

"I pride myself on associating with innovators in the medical field. When we combine forces we can make things happen that really move the needle on people's health and wellness. My science and research collaborations with Dr. She have been and continue to be productive in bringing solutions to patients. With this book he has brought the ancient teachings of TAO into play with Western Medicine. It is a great read and full of practical, efficacious tips for anyone who wants to extend their healthspan."

NAD has by virtue of its best laboratory science and clinical testing now found itself in the fast lane of anti-aging therapeutics

Dr She of Jinfiniti Precision Medicine has significant expertise in both the clinical lab and also in observing actual human data on individuals supplementing with this natural substance. His observations and analysis in this new book are well worth reading. Live long and well. "

Dr. Ron Klatz, MD, DL
President and Founder American Academy of Anti-Aging Medicine (A4M)

"As a pioneer in stem cells, platelet-rich plasma (PRP), and regenerative medicine, I have witnessed the remarkable evolution of Western medicine into high-tech realms unimaginable when I began my career as an orthopedic surgeon. Yet, amidst this rapid progress, it is vital to honor the wisdom of the past. Dr. She masterfully bridges ancient TAO philosophy with cutting-edge science and technology, creating a program that harmonizes timeless principles with modern innovation. This book is an invaluable guide for anyone striving for holistic health, vitality, and a long, vibrant life."

Dr. Joseph Purita
Pioneer in the use of Stem Cell and Platelet Rich Plasma for orthopaedic conditions. Inspector and proctor of surgeons in the use of lasers in arthroscopic and orthopaedic surgery. Star of the Super Beets commercials

---

"NAD levels decline during aging, and the only way to know if or how it can be reversed is through regular NAD quantification. With that in mind, NAD quantification with Jinfiniti is essential to my goal of minimizing disease risk, slowing aging and potentially, maximizing lifespan."

Dr. Michael Lustgarten
PhD. Nutrition and Aging Scientist, Tufts University, Conquer Aging or Die Trying YouTube Channel

---

"Monitoring intracellular NAD levels has been revolutionary in my clinical practice. I strongly recommend all my patients that struggle with low energy to get their intracellular NAD levels measured. The Jinfiniti NAD test is a game changer in my practice."

Dr. Edwin Lee
M.D., Renowned anti-aging doctor and speaker, Founder of Institute for Hormonal Balance, Orlando

---

AUTHOR'S PREFACE

"The Tao gives us life but does not claim to own us. It is ever acting on our behalf but expects nothing in return. It is our true guide but does not control us. Its presence is deep within the heart of every being."

—Loa-Tzu, *Tao Te Ching*

In this book, you will read in-depth discussions of recent scientific discoveries that can significantly improve people's lives. But it is not a love tome to science. I have been a scientist for more than 40 years. As a molecular biologist, I have often "geeked out" over revelations hidden in arcane data. But as my Ph. D. degree reminds me, I am a "doctor of philosophy." So, as a philosopher, I am a "lover of knowledge," and I welcome verifiable knowledge from every quarter. Moreover, inspired as I am by recent discoveries, I am not so enthralled in this present scientific moment that I am ready to discard knowledge that has stood the test of time. In fact, I view the current fad of "presentism," that tendency to divest contemporary culture of all thought that conflicts with current norms and perspectives, to be dangerously shortsighted.

There is much in our past that is worthy of preservation and rediscovery.

As a scientist, I value measurable and testable observations, whether they come from laboratory experiments or the cycles of nature. As a philosopher, I have found that truths never contradict each other. Rather, they augment and supplement one another. This is the symbiotic relationship I hope to present in this book.

At its heart, this book is a primer on human potential. It examines the current science of wellness and longevity, while drawing heavily on ancient wisdom which has guided seekers of truth for millennia. Thus, this book can be read as a guide for becoming more fully and deeply human.

Finally, I have always thought that science should be at service to mankind, not the other way around. Consistent with that attitude, I have refrained from using any tools of artificial intelligence to compose this book. I present it as a human-to-human conversation that I hope will engage your mind and also open your heart to your fullest potential.

INTRODUCTION

"The Tao that can be Told is not the True Tao;
Names that can be Named are not true Names."

—Lao-Tzu, *Tao Te Ching*

If you have picked up this book, you have doubtless heard something intriguing about NAD. Perhaps you have heard firsthand from a patient whose complaints of fatigue, sleeplessness, or mental fog miraculously vanished, or a healthcare provider has told you about possible benefits for your energy, mood, and longevity, or maybe you've seen advertisements from one of the many suppliers of NAD supplements promising The Fountain of Youth. Let me assure you that your interest in NAD has placed you on a profound path that can lead to optimized health for a lengthier lifespan, or what we call an extended healthspan.

Unfortunately, with every alleged panacea, we always find a swirl of misinformation, where anecdotal results are presented as norms and magical thinking usurps the role of hard science. Hopeful patients making their earnest health journey can fall under the dark cloud of hucksterism, where they overpay for products that fail to deliver the promised results, thus missing the opportunity for an optimized healthspan. This is a sad reality which this book hopes to combat.

The ancients of China had a concept of Self-Cultivation leading to inner peace, harmony with nature, and a longer, healthier life. They called this concept the *Tao*, which can be translated as The Way. In Chapter 14 of the *Tao Te Ching*, the philosopher Lao-Tzu explains:

Look,
And you never can see it—
It is too Subtle.

Listen,
And you never can hear it—
It is too Faint.

Feel for it,
And you never can take hold of it—
It is too Elusive.

The ancients understood that Self-Cultivation could not be achieved by striving, contending, competing; accumulating wealth, power, or fame; or rigorously studying from books. Quiet, solitude, and inaction were the keys to discerning the *Tao*.

Similarly, aggressive methods of enhancing NAD through whole NAD supplements and intravenous injections have not resulted in optimized cellular levels of NAD and so have not delivered the sought-after health benefits. Diet, exercise, and other lifestyle modifications are always good but do not 'help nature along' sufficiently to raise cellular NAD, which naturally declines with age.

Like the *Tao*, NAD optimization is elusive. The means for achieving optimization are subtle. But we are fortunate to live in an age where the mysteries of our human cells, those building blocks of life, are opening up to us. Molecular biologists, such as myself, have a greater understanding of the chemical processes taking place on a microscopic scale throughout the body, determining how much energy we have, how well we fight disease, and ultimately how long we might live.

Because of my background as a cellular biologist, I know what molecules to test for, I have developed tools to take precise measurements, along with effective methods to supplement essential compounds for optimal health. In short, our approach takes the guesswork out of diagnosing suboptimal conditions and provides targeted remedies that deliver impressive results. If you want to know why you fatigue easily, why you struggle with stubborn weight you cannot lose, why you sleep poorly, why you are not getting results at the gym, …and on and on, the reasons are measurable. You don't have to settle for vague platitudes and peps talks; it is possible to get a full explanation, based on your microbiology, along with a program of optimization that is specific to your individual needs.

In this book, I share my insights, based on hard science, about myriad issues related to NAD. You will learn the role of NAD in cell processes that impact the human healthspan, the consequences of age-related decline in NAD, and most importantly, the most efficient means of restoring optimal levels. This is the *Tao of NAD*, a path of Self-Cultivation that can enrich your life with greater energy, improved resistance to disease, a higher level of emotional peace, and a longer life. So, without further delay, let us begin.

CHAPTER 1

MY JOURNEY OF MANY THOUSANDS OF MILES

"When the best leader's work is done, the people say we did it ourselves."

—Lao-Tzu, *Tao Te Ching*

By now you might be wondering, "Who is this man who claims to know so much about NAD? How can he claim special knowledge that other healthcare providers and supplement manufacturers don't also have? How can he claim to know secrets about optimizing NAD levels that are not generally known?" These are fair questions, and you are prudent to ask. Allow me to give you a quick sketch of my background.

I was born in 1962 in rural China, in the province of Hubei. This is an area of central China, which Westerners would probably call "the middle of nowhere," except that its capital city, Wuhan, has recently gained unfortunate notoriety. My parents were subsistence farmers, working less than an acre of land to support my five sisters and me, their youngest. Although my parents were illiterate, they valued education for their children and saw that we received an education, even though the local schools were not very good. Despite our poverty, we were generally happy, because there was much love in our home. However, two unhappy incidents colored my childhood and would have an influence on my life decisions. An older sister died very young at 36, and my dad had a significant health scare with liver fibrosis when I was just 12 years old. That disease almost killed him. So, at a young age, I understood how important it was to have reliable healthcare. I also knew that our poverty was a barrier to getting that care and that reality struck me as terribly unjust.

During my childhood, China experienced its "Cultural Revolution," a turbulent ten-year period during which the Communist Party attempted to strengthen its control over society by purging remnants of capitalism and traditions that stood in the way of "progress." Many institutions drew criticism, including higher education, resulting in the closure of universities throughout the country. But with the death of Mao Zedong in 1976, the Cultural Revolution ended, and the universities were reopened in 1977. This was just in time for me, at age 16, to apply for admission.

In China, there was a national competition for university admission. Although I knew my high school education was of poor quality, I was determined to do well on the test, so I studied intensively for a couple of months prior. I felt the odds were against me, because not only was I competing against classmates who I thought were smarter than I, but older students who had been denied admission during the years of closure were also competing for spots. To gain entry, one needed a score of 280 points.

Several weeks after the testing, we got word of my score. I'd garnered 284 points and had won admission to the Huazhong University of Agriculture. My family was overjoyed for me. In fact, the entire community viewed my admission as a great honor. I thought that luck had played a key role because I could easily have scored five points lower and missed my chance. This element of luck hinted at a higher purpose for the education I was about to receive. But there was another lesson, one of attitude. I had applied myself for weeks in preparation, while some students who I thought were smarter had felt the weight of the odds against them and had not studied diligently.

So, as I prepared to enter university in the fall of 1978, I had mixed feelings. I knew that my poor high school education would initially be an impediment, but I was also confident that if I applied myself, I could succeed. I was buoyed by the support my family and community had given me, and I wanted to learn something useful for their benefit.

I majored in Aquaculture, which is the study of "fish farming." This might seem odd, since my province is landlocked, but fishing in the lakes and rivers is an important part of the local economy and sustenance for many poor families. This course of study introduced me to fish biology, which focused on raising healthier, more abundant stocks of fish. A key factor was fish genetics, which influenced resistance to disease, growth rates, and the nutritional value of the fish. This study would lead to my interest in biotechnology as a way to increase productivity and quality.

If this field of study seems too esoteric, it's worth mentioning that some of my classmates are now living like kings on the riches they earned improving fish farming in central China.

One of the common misconceptions about China is that personal wealth is forbidden under the Communist system. But even though the Communist Party does exercise significant control over the industrial sectors it deems critical to the population, the Party also recognizes that individuals need incentives to be productive. Thus, since 1978, China has become more capitalistic, at least economically, and entrepreneurs with drive and vision have become quite wealthy.

At any rate, my college studies ran their course, and I was ready to return home with my degree. In my heart, I yearned for my family and wanted to help my parents, especially now that they were getting older. Duty to family is an important value in China, which had been bred into my brain. I was therefore resolved to be a farmer, working my small patch of land. Fortunately, an older, wiser classmate set me on a different path.

It was right around the time of the Lunar New Year, which is a lengthy holiday festival in China. People from all over the country take off from work and travel to their home provinces to enjoy two weeks of festivities. I had a friend from my hometown who was studying at another school, and we had planned that he would come to my university, and we would travel home together. But before he arrived, I had a conversation that changed my life.

I mentioned earlier that because the universities had been closed for so long, there were older students on my level. I had confided to one of these older men that I would go back to the farm and work with my father. He told me I was crazy. Then he explained in very logical terms that the help I could give my family as a farmer was sorely limited, especially since I'm small in stature and manual labor is not my forte. However, the help I could give my parents as a career professional was potentially unlimited. Not only that, but I might make scientific discoveries that could help my entire community. These contributions would far outweigh any good I could do raising turnips.

My older friend had me convinced, so I decided I would spend the Lunar New Year break at school, studying for the graduate school exam. When my hometown friend arrived at my dorm, I told him, "Sorry, dude. Have a nice trip, but I'm staying." I felt bad because he'd gone out of his way to fetch me, but my course was set.

There were not many grad school choices open to me, where I could continue my study of fish farming. However, the Chinese government offered scholarships for study in the United States that would focus on fish pathology. I decided to compete for a spot, and again my older, wiser friend told me I was crazy. The competition would be intense, and students from better universities in the big cities would have the inside track. I should mention here that although my school in Huazhong ranks in the top 50 of Chinese colleges today, it was not highly regarded back then. I would be a "hick from the sticks" competing against savvy "city slickers." But I would not be deterred. I studied intensively and very nervously took the exam.

When the results came in, I found I had scored highest on the exam by one hundred points! This victory added greatly to my confidence, to the point where I would never again think that a task cannot be done. No matter how difficult a problem might seem, I only ask whether it must be done. If the answer is yes, I always believe I can find a way.

So, as I held the notice in my hand, I was thinking, "USA, here I come!" But the scholarship board had other plans. For reasons that were never explained, they switched my foreign study program to France. This made little difference to me since I couldn't speak English or French, and for this hick from the sticks, any international travel was bound to be an adventure.

It was 1983 when I journeyed to Montpellier in France for a crash course in the French language at the university. Montpellier is a beautiful city in the south, close to the Mediterranean Sea, but I didn't have much time to enjoy it. After a couple of months, I was off to L'Institut national polytechnique de Toulouse, the National Polytechnic Institute of Toulouse. This was another lovely city, with majestic views of the snow-capped Pyrenees mountains in the west. I spent one school year there, earning a master's degree in Cytogenetics, that is, cell genetics.

After Toulouse, I returned to l'université de Montpellier, this time studying molecular biology and population genetics. At that time, molecular biology was a new field of study, and I felt this was the future. Cells, after all, are the building blocks of organisms, and molecules are the building blocks of cells. If I could master molecular tools, I could do anything in biology and medicine. If I could optimize cellular health, then tissue, organ, and systemic health would surely follow. This was also my introduction to quantitative science, analyzing mountains of data to answer biological questions.

These days, there is almost an obsession with "Big Data" in virtually every human endeavor, from the economy and commerce to social media and entertainment to health science. In my studies at Montpellier, we married data gathered at the cellular level to qualitative analysis. So, almost 40 years ago, I was at the forefront of Big Data, exploring questions that are now being addressed through artificial intelligence.

I believe my Montpellier training distinguishes me from many biologists who have not developed a "quantitative mind." This missing trait prevents them from designing tests that can produce actionable data and creates blind spots that prevent them from analyzing data in an insightful manner that opens up new discoveries. The long-term impact on my career was a deeper understanding of methodology and the proper way to approach scientific experimentation. In population genetics, we connect a lot of data, and on the surface, the meaning of the data might not be apparent. The human mind is not able to figure out the meaning of such complex data unless we use computational tools designed to bring to light the underlying principles hidden in the data. Thus, in our experiments, we were doing elementary AI (artificial intelligence) to understand what the data meant and what it could teach us.

My Montpellier experience profoundly shaped how I conduct research and gave me a great appreciation for the value of data gathered through testing. Data empowers us to take action, but it also enables us to monitor processes and measure results.

In 1987, after three and a half years of study, I earned a PhD in Molecular and Population Genetics at Montpellier. But there was a major difference in my coursework. To graduate, I needed to complete one research project, which involved a continuation of my studies of fish genetics. However, I had developed an interest in mitochondria function, and I thought important knowledge would be gained by delving into this subject. Briefly, mitochondria are organelles; they are subcellular structures, which perform specific tasks within a cell, much like an organ that services the body. The nucleus of the cell is also an organelle. Interestingly, although we find most of our DNA—the strands that contain our genetic code—in the nucleus, we also have mitochondrial DNA. I was intrigued by what I knew about DNA and wanted to learn more. I learned, for example, that while nuclear DNA is inherited from both parents, mitochondrial DNA is only passed through the mother, which is an interesting phenomenon.

In the mid-1980s, this area of molecular biology was new, since researchers had only started developing tools to study DNA and RNA in the 1970s. I wanted to master the new tools that were coming out, but those were not available to study fish, only mice. So, I worked on a second research project in mouse genetics, and I'm very glad I did. Forty years ago, we didn't know how important mitochondrial functions are. Today, we know the mitochondria drive cellular energy production and thus promote overall cell health and longevity.

Having received my PhD, I needed to make a career decision. I couldn't remain a student forever, or could I? I wanted to continue studying molecular biology, especially since a new method of testing was about to revolutionize what we could do to study DNA. I am referring to the Polymerase Chain Reaction, or PCR, test. You no doubt recognize the initials from the test used to diagnose COVID-19 infection during the pandemic. But you probably don't realize what a major step forward this test was for molecular biology.

The problem, simply put, is that if you want to study DNA, you need almost an infinite number of identical strands. You cannot obtain these millions or even billions of strands from a natural source. You need a reliable method for propagating identical DNA strands, or as we say, amplifying DNA. For the process to work, you need a reagent, i.e., a compound that can facilitate the process. That's what the term polymerase refers to; this is any enzyme that catalyzes the synthesis of DNA. Each time through a process of temperature changes, heating and then cooling, the DNA doubles. Eventually, if the process works, you'll have a sufficient amount of DNA for experimentation. But there were a couple of problems.

First, it was a slow, manual process consisting of countless cycles over many, many hours. In our lab, we had to take samples from one water bath to another to affect the temperature change up to forty times. Second, the reagent might break down and become incapable of catalyzing, so the process would stall. So, scientists had to find an enzyme that not only could work but could remain stable for a long series of cycles. This search led to the discovery of Taq DNA polymerase in the late 1970s.

Long story short, a researcher named Kary Mullis created the PCR process for exponentially amplifying DNA in 1983 and published his findings in 1985. It wasn't long before machines automated the process to spare researchers endless hours of transferring samples by hand from one water bath to another.

Now that tedious downtime had been removed from the process, this area of molecular biology was set to take off. I wanted to pursue this line of scientific inquiry, but in 1987 it was so new that few universities offered the opportunity to do PCR-related study. (Mullis and a colleague would eventually receive the Nobel Prize in Chemistry, but not until 1993.) Only two laboratories in the world were doing the work, and not very well. I was fortunate to find an opening for post-doctoral studies in molecular biology at the University of Florida, starting in January 1988. My mentor was one of the very few scientists doing PCR-related studies, and he was as determined as I was to master the technology.

PCR testing is helpful for a huge range of problems: medical diagnostics, screening donated blood for pathogens, crime scene forensics, detecting food-borne pathogens, and analyzing ancient fossils. My work at the University of Florida had a very gratifying application. I was primarily involved in research for new testing methods to match tissue and organ donors with recipients.

We received a major grant to apply PCR technology to HLA typing, to match tissues and organs more precisely. HLA refers to human leukocyte antigens, which are proteins found in most of the body's cells. The immune system uses these proteins as markers to distinguish our own cells from the cells of an invader, such as a viral or bacterial infection. If a surgical team were to transplant an organ into a host with incompatible HLA, the immune system would attack the organ as it would an infection, and the organ would fail. We had our first clinical diagnostic test in the early 1990s. It was gratifying to know that our work would extend the lives of so many people who needed a new organ, bone marrow, or cord blood to survive.

I remained in Florida until 2002 when I moved on to Augusta Medical College of Georgia (now Augusta University), where I am currently engaged. Most of my time has been spent in research, but I've done some teaching for graduate students. I continued to work in areas that have immediate medical applications, but I transitioned from life-saving medical diagnostics to preventative medical research. This mostly means identifying risk factors that lead to disease in the future. Initially, going back to my days in Florida, I studied Type I diabetes, trying to understand the molecular and environmental factors. During this time, I actually discovered the gene related to Type I diabetes. The goal of this research was to identify high-risk individuals and come up with precise approaches for preventing symptoms and full-blown disease. So, instead of correcting a bad situation, as with organ matching, the goal was to prevent bad things from happening. There is a bit of the *Tao* in this thinking, because as Lao Tzu would say, "That which is at peace is easily maintained." In other words, an ounce of prevention is worth a pound of cure.

At first, I examined Type I diabetes in children. Then I explored the condition as an age-related illness. Since diabetes is a disease of the whole body, our work covered everything from genetics to biochemistry, cellular biology, social behavior, psychological effects, and related diseases, such as neuropathy. We even looked at the social and economic impact of diabetes. This gave me a great appreciation of how outside forces shape behaviors that invite disease, and how this can happen on the grand scale we see here in the United States today. Diabetes is often naturally occurring, because there is a genetic component, but it can be induced through poor diet, a sedentary lifestyle, psychological stress, and emotional trauma. It is also a disease that progresses as we age, and which prematurely ages our bodily systems.

The study of disease naturally led me to longevity, because I was asking so many questions about how people could live healthily longer than they were. I wondered whether, if we could prevent diabetes, we could prevent other age-related diseases. Could we identify the risk factors for premature aging? And modify lifestyles to mitigate the risks before the onset of disease?

As you might know, the root causes of diabetes overlap in a major way with the root causes of cardiovascular disease, which is also age-related. A high-sugar diet, a sedentary lifestyle, smoking, and alcohol consumption are all factors that contribute to diabetes as well as cardiovascular disease.

Of course, many people have addressed these illnesses from a lifestyle angle. I wanted to explore the issues on the cellular level. What we found was micronutrient deficiency. In other words, cells were malnourished and therefore were less capable of performing the functions necessary for producing energy, reproducing, healing, and contributing to the larger functions of the organs. As a result, cells were "winding down," bodily systems became sluggish, and the aches and pains we associated with advanced age were becoming more and more common.

The micronutrient deficiency we observed pointed us towards NAD. Scientists had first discovered this natural compound in human cells in 1906, but it has taken more than a century for us to begin to appreciate its significance. We shall cover this in a subsequent chapter but suffice to say now, NAD has been a revelation. It is almost as if all my previous training had led me to this one moment. I recall that fateful decision to study for graduate school rather than return to the farm for Lunar New Year, and I suspect that I finally know how I can do the most good for the most people. It is in helping them optimize their NAD for their greatest possible healthspan.

Allow me to backtrack for a couple of paragraphs, because in all the excitement of relating the events of my professional life, I've neglected to mention that I got married in 1994. While in Florida, I met a lovely woman, a nurse who was also engaged in real estate sales. We fell in love, got married, and eventually had three children. Unfortunately, our relationship faltered due to mutual workaholism and a difference in philosophies. We initiated the divorce in 2012, which wasn't finalized until 2015.

Divorce was a horrible experience. I give it zero stars and cannot recommend. It left me feeling totally depleted. In my body, my spirit, and my checking account. But it left me free to pursue my goal of forming my biotech company. Shortly thereafter, I met the woman who became my second wife. And as the song says, "Love is lovelier, the second time around." As a couple, we are much more compatible. She is a PhD scientist, who has been extremely important to *Jinfiniti* and was instrumental in developing our test for intracellular NAD. We have two wonderful children together.

But you can probably imagine that with the emotional highs and lows and the constant research work, ol' Jin was burning his candle at both ends and in the middle. I started to spiral down, developing the types of aches and pains you'd expect in a much older man. Perhaps the best way to illustrate what was happening—and how NAD brought me back—is through my tennis game.

I became enamored of tennis in my twenties, and it soon became my favorite means of exercise. But starting in my late thirties, post-workout soreness became a real issue. Then pre-workout stiffness. It got to the point where I had to take

Tylenol before a game, or I wouldn't recover for weeks. But even with Tylenol, I had to warm up for thirty minutes before I felt loose enough to participate. Eventually, due to wrist, shoulder, back, and knee pain, I could only play tennis once a week. When I moved to Georgia in 2002, I started taking prescription drugs for knee pain. I also had such bad sciatica that I couldn't sit down on the couch at the end of the day.

But after three months of optimizing my NAD, all of that pain went away. I didn't even need Tylenol to play tennis. I didn't need to warm up and I didn't tire out.

I should also add that I developed asthma and terrible seasonal allergies. I took medications for these maladies for twenty years. But one day, maybe six months after I started my NAD supplementation, I appeared as a guest on the Marcel James podcast. We were discussing the benefits of NAD, when he said his allergies had disappeared. I realized at that moment that I hadn't been taking my meds. My allergies had vanished a few months earlier and I hadn't even noticed!

Now let's talk about a few more benefits I have personally experienced. Not to sound boastful, but my bedroom performance has improved dramatically. That's right: I sleep much more deeply and soundly, and I awaken fully restored. But if you were thinking of sexual performance, I'll modestly admit, that's improved, too. For most people in their sixties, a declining sex drive or frustrations in performance become issues. Not for folks on NAD.

My liver function has improved, as verified by the presence of liver enzymes and reduced levels of triglycerides. My inflammatory biomarkers have improved, which is no surprise, given the absence of pain. My skin has more moisture to it and looks younger. At a recent Lunar New Year party, several old friends said I had become so much younger. Honestly, I haven't really aged the last few years, but my classmates certainly have. As for mental clarity, which can create uncertainty and distress for older adults, my cognitive functions remain very strong. There's been no noticeable decline.

Altogether, I feel like a totally different person from who I was before NAD. And I continue to feel better and better. I made the mistake of stopping the supplement once for nine days, and I noticed the difference. NAD really is the key to a more vibrant, pain-free life.

But it's not enough for me to feel younger, more energetic, and pain free. I wish the same for you!

I have always wanted my learning to serve others, starting with that 'bred in the brain' notion of repaying my parents. Perhaps because I saw my parents work so hard to care for our family, my focus has been on helping people who want to help themselves. If you are reading this book, you probably fall into that category. And I welcome you on this journey I call the *Tao of NAD*.

But be aware: it is you more than I who will be responsible for what follows. I can gather all the empirical data imaginable and present it as clearly as possible. But ultimately, only you can do the work to optimize your NAD for greater healthspan. I can provide information, but you must follow the *Tao of NAD*, just as Lao Tzu's students followed the *Tao Te Ching*. You must commit to the course and 'walk the walk.' Then, when you have fully optimized your cellular NAD, and you are living the benefits, I will be happy to hear you say that you did it yourself.

CHAPTER 2

THE ETERNAL TRUTH OF THE TAO

"Therefore: In dwelling, choose modest quarters, in thinking, value stillness, in dealing with others, be kind, in choosing words, be sincere, in leading, be just, in working, be competent, in acting, choose the correct timing. Follow these words and there will be no error."

Lao Tzu, *Tao Te Ching*

Before we explore the *Tao of NAD*, it will be helpful to understand the original *Tao Te Ching*, attributed to the ancient Chinese philosopher Lao-Tzu, who lived in the 6th century B.C.E. This was the end of the Iron Age and the beginning of Classical Antiquity. Society, technology, and knowledge were primitive, and warfare was fairly constant, due to a xenophobic fear of foreigners and the notion that conquest was a legitimate means of nation-building. No one lived by the Golden Rule, except for the version that says, "He who has the gold makes the rules." As a result, life was, as the English philosopher Thomas Hobbs would later describe it, "solitary, poor, nasty, brutish, and short." Yet, everywhere, philosophers, prophets, and scholars sought solutions for the ills of the world.

In China, the ancient philosophers drew clues for how mankind should behave from nature. In nature, they observed harmonious cycles and long periods of homeostasis. Of course, there were times when nature would pitch a fit. Great storms and floods, fires, and earthquakes made their mark. But nature would always return to its cycle: spring rains, summer crops, fall harvests, and winter hibernation.

For Lao-Tzu, much of the strife in human existence came from men contending against one another, competing for fame, striving for glory, and seeking dominance. This focus on external power led to cruelty, sorrow, waste, illness, and death. Lao-Tzu wanted to lead people off the path of destruction predicated on abusive power to the quiet, harmony, balance, and health characterized by inner power.

His seminal work, *Tao Te Ching* can be translated as the *Path to Inner Power*. In this collection of philosophical musings in verse, Lao-Tzu explains that people cannot attain inner power by striving, competing, accumulating, exerting, vanquishing, defeating, and dominating. Instead, true inner power comes from inner peace, which one gains through inactivity, simplicity, humility, yielding, waiting, and resting.

Lao-Tzu relies on three main images to illustrate the apparent paradox of inner power: water, the valley, and the uncarved block of wood. Of water, Lao Tzu writes:

> *Water is fluid, soft, and yielding. But water will wear away rock, which is rigid and cannot yield. As a rule, whatever is fluid, soft,*

> *and yielding will overcome whatever is rigid and hard. This is another paradox: what is soft is strong.*

The source of water's strength is its humility:

> *All streams flow to the sea because it is lower than they are. Humility gives it its power. If you want to govern the people, you must place yourself below them. If you want to lead the people, you must learn how to follow them.*

The ocean does not strive to become mightier than the rivers that feed it. It amasses its strength through inactivity, by placing itself below the sources that flow into it.

Similarly, the valley becomes fertile by waiting and abiding. Lao-Tzu describes the Taoists of Old as "broad and open as a valley. They were empty, not craving honor and fame. They embraced all." Lao-Tzu describes the freedom of enlightenment as a form of openness:

> *We wait for whatever comes, as a valley welcomes the river. To notice this enlightenment, we sit patiently and wait, as for mud to settle and our minds to become clear. Life then lives itself in us.*

All worldly striving and contending puts pressure on the human person and causes division. It sets the people against one another, as in war, but it also sets a single person against himself. The *Tao*, on the other hand, makes a person whole again. Lao-Tzu writes:

> *Know honor, yet keep humility. Be the valley of the universe! Being the valley of the universe, ever true and resourceful, return to the state of the uncarved block.*

The uncarved block is a metaphor for unity, integrity, and peace. Through periods of rest and humble reflection, we can recover our original state, the balance we enjoyed before all the striving and contending fractured our mind and ruined our health.

Of course, the problems that Lao-Tzu observed in his time are still with us. Our modern technological society has placed everything at our fingertips except inner peace. We strive and contend to make a living and build a career. We compete for better positions and higher pay. We comfort ourselves by acquiring the newest fashions and consumer gadgets, but this is a distraction, not true comfort. And, given today's social media, everyone can seek some glory or fame, just by making posts and collecting 'likes.'

What we do not do is contemplate nature, observing its signs, to imitate the harmony found there. If anything, modern humanity lives contrary to nature, seeking to conquer it, rather than draw peace from it. Yet, attempting to conquer nature is a fool's errand. Firstly, because there is so much that is unknowable, and secondly, because we are natural beings, and conflict with nature invariably places us in conflict with ourselves.

Truly, our society gives us ample opportunity to divide—to fracture—ourselves and withdraw from those around us. This leads to a host of symptoms, including anxiety, depression, fatigue, inflammation, chronic pain, sleeplessness, mental fogginess, and early aging. We cannot live like this; we must find harmony, peace, and health. We must return to the uncarved block.

CHAPTER 3

FROM THE PILLARS OF THE SKY TO THE PILLARS OF THE TAO

"The nameless uncarved block
Is but freedom from desire,
And I if I cease to desire and remain still,
The empire will be at peace of its own accord."

Lao Tzu, *Tao Te Ching*

Like other ancient cultures, China developed a mythology drawn from the landscape and nature. Like other cultures, the Chinese observed the separation between the world below and the firmament above and saw mountains as pillars holding up the sky as well as staircases ascending to the heavens. In Chinese mythology, there were eight such mountain pillars, located in the cardinal directions. Some were based on actual mountains; others were wholly imaginary. In time, these mountain pillars came to represent virtues, which made men upright and allowed them to ascend toward a more perfect state of being. Eventually, philosophers began to speak in terms of "Pillars" of Confucianism and of the *Tao*.

While there is no universally agreed-upon list of *Pillars of the Tao*, there are qualities and practices that are considered essential, and writers will off-and-on refer to these as pillars. I believe that the most salient points of the *Tao* include:

- **SELF-CULTIVATION** — The *Tao* is a path of self-development and requires a conscious, disciplined effort at self-improvement through the practices Lao-Tzu and other teachers have described.
- **HUMILITY** — A bedrock principle of the *Tao*, humility prevents an individual from seeking fame, glory, and exalted position. It prevents fruitless activity, based entirely on ambition rather than necessity. It prevents contending and competition, which divides one person against another. Humility also deters us from pursuing disagreements which then escalate into costly confrontations.
- **NON-ACTION** — With this concept, the Taoists recognize the need to refrain from busy-body activity and overly ambitious, highly exertive tasks. The body and spirit can only be taxed so far before we need a respite. Taoists advise us to withdraw, meditate, and "return to the uncarved block" to restore our natural state of inner peace.
- **FREEDOM FROM DESIRE** — Human nature prompts us to seek satisfaction for a wide range of desires. Whether it's rich food, wine, succulent desserts, riches, fame, or sexual pleasure, pursuing these desires too zealously invariably leads to frustration, disappointment, and internal strife. We can develop addictions, becoming a mere pawn of our desires. The Taoists stress self-mastery,

because only by conquering our desires can we free our bodies and minds.

- **FRUGALITY** — A Taoist should be content with less, rather than laboring exhaustively to be able to spend lavishly.
- **SIMPLICITY** — As with humility and frugality, this virtue protects individuals from the wasteful toil and divisiveness that arises from great ambition and avarice.
- **BALANCE AND UNITY** — In Chinese philosophy, the rhythm and cycles of nature operate under the complementary principles of Yin and Yang. Yin is the quiet, female, intuitive force associated with the earth. The earth receives from the heavens and gives forth new life, giving mankind the food we need to survive. Yang is the strong, male, creative force associated with the heavens above. The motion of the heavens brings about change on earth, as rainfall yields vegetation. Neither force is better than the other; each is essential. The optimal state of our physical universe is a balance of Yin and Yang. This balance is also essential for individual health.

A person who follows the *Tao* is also said to obtain other virtues, such as propriety, honor, loyalty, benevolence, righteousness, integrity, justice, love, harmony, peace, and a healthy sense of shame.

These principles have survived thousands of years because they are founded upon a true understanding of the human condition, about what makes us tick and what can bring that ticking to an abrupt and sad stop. The ancient *Pillars of the Tao* are still relevant today. But since we have deeper insights into human nature, especially on the cellular level, it is possible to update the *Tao* for our time.

In the coming chapters, I shall attempt to present an optimized *Tao*, made possible by recent scientific discoveries related to NAD.

CHAPTER 4

THE PROBLEM OF MODERN LIVING AND THE NEED FOR A NEW TAO

"Too much brightness blinds the eyes. Too much sound deafens the ears. Too much flavor ruins the tongue. Chasing desires to excess turns your mind towards madness, and valuing precious things impairs good judgment."

Lao-Tzu, *Tao Te Ching*

Many problems that plagued the ancients are virtually unknown to us. Yes, there are still corners of the world where clean, running water is unavailable, wood to fire a stove is scarce, and the lack of antibiotics can turn a small cut into a life-threatening wound. But we who live in the developed world suffer more from abundance than from want. We suffer from our displacement from nature and from the paradoxical reality that technology designed to make our lives more comfortable often makes life unbearable. We force ourselves to conform to abnormal norms which rob us of peace and diminish our health. Here are just a few problems our modern society has created.

Poor Diet

Where to begin with this dilemma? There is no shortage of food in the developed world, but choices made by industries and individual consumers have resulted in widespread malnutrition. Of course, you wouldn't immediately think the public was malnourished, because so many are obese. Yet, two apparently contradictory facts can be true at the same time. But why is it so?

On the industry side, agribusiness has introduced genetically modified foods, processed foods, and artificial ingredients into the "food stream." This has been done to increase yields, prolong shelf-life, and entice consumers to eat more of the product. But the health consequences for consumers have been horrendous. According to the Center for Food Safety[1], GMO foods present six key risks to consumers: toxicity, allergic reactions, antibiotic resistance, immuno-suppression, cancer, and loss of nutrition. Food writer Mark Bittmas has warned that since food is defined as "a substance that provides nutrition and promotes growth," and poison as "a substance that promotes illness," then "much of what is produced by industrialized agriculture is, quite literally, not food but poison." This problem extends to "food products" sold as organic and made with all-natural ingredients. These can still qualify as processed poisons, not because of what has gone into them, but for what has been done to them.

---

1 *https://www.centerforfoodsafety.org/issues/311/ge-foods/ge-food-and-your-health*

You might ask what the U.S. Department of Agriculture and the U.S. Food and Drug Administration is doing about this problem. How can government regulators be fully aware of the dangers of processed foods, yet do nothing to protect the public? Unfortunately, the priority for these government agencies is commerce, not public health. Dr. Robert H. Lustig, an American pediatric endocrinologist, famous for promoting metabolic health and combatting the epidemic of childhood obesity, takes a jaundiced view of the situation. He believes that Big Food's processed diet is designed to make us sick, so more consumers will require drugs sold by Big Pharma.

We should briefly note that industrial agriculture is also an ecological disaster. Farmland is overutilized, leading to depleted soil, which industrial farms fortify with chemical fertilizers. Such fertilizers can increase crop yields but do not enhance the nutritional quality of the food. Thus, we wind up with a glut of practically worthless food. Moreover, soil runoff from industrial farms can have a deleterious effect on waterways and marine life.

On the consumer side, people make food choices based on faulty criteria, such as taste, convenience, and easy availability. We give little thought to nutrition, especially if a nutritious meal requires us to go out of our way to purchase fresh ingredients and spend more than a couple of minutes zapping the meal in a microwave. We also center too many activities around eating, especially sedentary activities, such as watching television.

The result is a widespread crisis of metabolic dysfunction, afflicting about 88 percent of Americans. Our deadly combination of poor nutrition, overweight, and inactivity gives rise to a plethora of health issues, including diabetes, hypertension, coronary heart disease, stroke, gallbladder disease, osteoarthritis, sleep apnea, fatigue, chronic pain due to inflammation, and a variety of cancers. People in this physical state have a low quality of life, often exacerbated by mental health issues, such as depression and anxiety.

In his research, Dr. Lustig has identified eight pathologies, which are our most common killers: heart disease, cancer, stroke, chronic lower respiratory disease, Alzheimer's disease, diabetes, influenza/pneumonia, and kidney disease. Notably, none of these conditions are curable via drugs. Only five respond to exercise, leading Dr. Lustig to conclude, "You can't outrun a bad diet."

The only therapy that makes a difference across all eight pathologies is a sound diet. Real food nourishes us on a metabolic level. That's because our bodies know what to do with real food. It breaks it down into assimilable vitamins and minerals, which convert into cellular food like NAD, thus increasing metabolic function.

"If you do not fix your food," Dr. Lustig warns, "you continue to court disease and untimely death. If we do not fix our food, we will continue to court societal and planetary oblivion."

Pollution in the Air and Water

Every so often, a story of catastrophic exposure to pollutants makes headlines. We read about a community, such as Love Canal, New York, Flint, Michigan, or Camp Lejeune, North Carolina. Or we hear how rescue workers who sifted through the smoldering rubble of the World Trade Center in 2001 are still developing deadly cancers twenty years later. But for the most part, we ignore pollution, counting it as a cost of modern living, overlooking the fact that it is a silent killer.

Unfortunately, in an industrial society, there will always be chemical waste, and not all of it can be contained. Workers in heavy industry and the mostly poor people living close to industrial centers suffer the worst exposure and can develop debilitating diseases. Residents of large cities must also contend with auto emissions creating blankets of smog. On "poor air quality days," our eyes may water and our nostrils and throats sting.

Chronic exposure to air pollution causes a variety of illnesses, including asthma, bronchitis, chronic obstructive pulmonary disease (COPD), cardiovascular diseases, cancers, neurological disorders, gastrointestinal disorders, kidney diseases, liver diseases, and skin diseases. Health issues related to water pollution include infectious diseases caused by pathogens (e.g., typhoid, giardiasis, encephalitis, and hepatitis), liver and kidney damage, neurological problems, reproductive issues including birth defects, and thyroid disorders.

On the positive side, countries are doing a much better job of regulating industrial waste and emissions than in the past. When the oil industry removed lead from gasoline in the 1970s, that was a major step forward for the environment and the human population. But we must do more because even low levels of exposure to pollutants can substantially diminish our health.

An Atomized Society

Community and a sense of belonging are essential for human flourishing, and unfortunately, we are losing these aspects of life. It is a sad irony that the more densely populated our urban areas become, the more those residents withdraw from their neighbors. Social isolation, as we saw vividly during the COVID lockdowns, can lead to many severe mental health issues, such as anxiety, depression, and hopelessness. An atomized society is a breeding ground for addiction, suicide, and all manners of anti-social behavior.

Human beings need meaningful, intimate contact with others. When we cannot relate to one another through normal channels, loneliness becomes a great burden, and we seek outlets through unhealthy practices, such as viewing pornography. Due to the Internet, people are being exposed to pornography at younger ages. A recent study[2] showed that 56.6 percent of students at a Catholic university reported being "lifetime" consumers and 13.5 percent admitted to "severe or extremely severe levels of depression, anxiety, and stress." The study concluded that "compulsive pornography use significantly affect[s] all three mental health parameters (depression, anxiety, and stress) in both sexes."

Other studies have concluded that viewing pornography can actually cause changes in the brain. Porn viewers can develop mental health issues that include high feelings of distress, anxiety episodes or generalized anxiety, emotional avoidance and detachment, feelings of loneliness, irritability, and anger. Excessive porn use has also been shown to decrease sexual

2 *https://www.ncbi.nlm.nih.gov/pmc/articles/PMC7835260/*

arousal, increase problems of sexual performance, and lower a person's sexual satisfaction. All of these issues create a downward spiral of loneliness, detachment, and hopelessness.

Overstimulated, Media-Driven, Consumer-Centric Living

When Lao-Tzu wrote that "too much brightness blinds the eyes," he could not have imagined the electronic images that bombard us almost everywhere we go. Whether it's television, computer screens, smartphones, or electronic billboards, there seems to be no escaping media and its constant demand that we "buy, buy, buy!" We're presented images of fashionable lifestyles and coveted possessions. We are pressured to pursue opulence, whatever the cost to our peace of mind, relationships, and physical health. If we fall short of the media's ideal, we're programmed to feel inadequacy and shame.

Few people realize that America's obsessive consumerism can be traced back to the machinations of one man: a public relations pioneer named Edward Louis Bernays. In the early 20th century, Bernays grasped that the field of psychology, which was intended to help people recover their mental health, could be used to manipulate human behavior on a grand scale. One notorious example was his work with the tobacco industry to double the market for cigarettes by inducing women to smoke. This was the time during which suffragettes were demanding the right for women to vote. Bernays branded cigarettes as "Torches of Freedom," and smoking as a sign of a liberated woman. Imagine selling an addictive substance that ruins one's health as a mark of freedom! How many untimely and painful deaths resulted from that manipulation? Advertisers today continue to use Bernays' methods to entice consumers to buy products they don't need and can't afford, many of which are ruinous to their health, all to conform to fabricated standards of glamor.

High-Stress Occupations

Perhaps the only thing worse than a dead-end job is one that drives us to an early death. Stress is another silent killer, which can ruin our health. According to the Centers for Disease Control[3], the early warning signs of job stress include frequent headaches, sleep disturbances, difficulty concentrating, irritability, short temper, and upset stomach. Prolonged stress can lead to debilitating illnesses, such as cardiovascular disease, musculoskeletal disorders (e.g., back and neck pain), ulcers, cancer, and impaired immune function leading to chronic sickness. Stress also increases the likelihood of a workplace accident, causing injury, and raises the risk of mental health problems, including depression, which can lead to suicide.

A few recent surveys indicate just how much stress American workers are under. A Northwestern Life survey found that 40 percent of workers reported their job is "very or extremely stressful." A survey by the Families and Work Institute found that 26 percent of workers are "often or very often burned out or stressed by their work." Finally, a Yale University study noted that 29 percent of workers feel "quite a bit or extremely stressed at work."

What causes stress on the job? Here are some of the leading factors:

- Overexertion

3 *https://www.cdc.gov/niosh/docs/99-101/default.html*

- Long hours
- Long commutes
- Low pay
- Rigid routines
- Overly demanding management
- Poor social environment in the workplace
- Lack of support from coworkers and supervisors
- Poorly defined and/or burdensome work roles
- Insecure employment

All of these issues are not just bad for employee health, they also hurt worker productivity. Some companies have come to realize that happy and relaxed workers serve the company's mission better. However, too many companies treat their workers with callous disregard, either because their leadership does not care or because they simply don't know how to change the culture of a large organization. As Lao-Tzu would say, "That journey of a thousand miles, starts with a single step." But that is a step too many companies are loathe to take.

Frantic Schedules With Poor Work/Life Balance

On top of high stress occupations, many individuals have demanding personal lives. You might be going to school at night or taking classes on weekends. You might have children, whose own busy schedules demand that you shuttle them to and from school and to various activities. You might be single and looking for a mate. You might be married and struggling to find time for your spouse. Hobbies, charitable work, community activism, and countless other concerns can keep you constantly on the go. During this time, you're running on pure adrenaline, or perhaps caffeine and sugar. But you cannot maintain this torrid pace forever, and one of these days, your body will tell you so.

Reliance on Medications to Overcome the Stresses of Unnatural Living

Lao-Tzu's prescription for the ailments of 21st-century living would be the *Tao*. Become the valley. Return to the uncarved block. However, the *Tao* requires a commitment to the process of self-cultivation. It requires a resetting of priorities and a re-ordering of our life. If instead, someone offers a pill to alleviate one or more symptoms, allowing us to maintain the patterns we've grown used to, we willingly take the pill. It's the easy way out; it makes fewer demands of us. Unfortunately, medicating symptoms rarely produce a cure. The underlying illness remains untreated, and soon new symptoms emerge, more debilitating than the last. So, we seek more pills. And on and on.

Western medicine (and thus Western society) has a pill problem. And it is getting more severe all the time. Partly, this is a natural outgrowth of highly beneficial science, but it is also an unfortunate perversion of good medicine in the service of corporate greed.

Perhaps because of Europe's experience of the Black Plague, and subsequent scourges, such as smallpox, Western scientists have almost exclusively focused on combating infectious diseases. This model of healthcare sees disease as the product of an outside invader attacking the body. The remedy is to destroy the invader with antivirals or antibiotics. Of course, this is a reasonable—and at times absolutely necessary—approach to infection and other acute illnesses.

But, as we know, what is essential is not always sufficient. Disease does not always occur because a particular virus or bacterium is potent; sometimes illness occurs because systems are worn out or deficient. People develop chronic illnesses because their lives are out of balance. Their body and mind lose health long before they come down sick.

Yet, Western medicine does not have an answer to chronic illness due to systemic imbalance and depletion. Treatments are heavily dependent on drugs to ease symptoms, sedate nerves, and numb pain. Often, these remedies come with dangerous side effects, which patients are told to accept as the cost of feeling better. Anyone who has ever listened to a prescription drug commercial on TV or radio has heard the long list of warnings that accompany the ad. For those of us who are not suffering from the targeted illness, the thought of risking the announced side effects fills us with trepidation. But the suffering patient willingly accepts the drug as their long-sought answer. And somewhere Edward Louis Bernays is smiling.

This brings us to the second point about our pill problem: pharmaceutical giants using direct-to-consumer (DTC) advertising to create a culture of pill-popping. Since the days of traveling snake oil salesmen, civil authorities have been wary of individuals and corporations bypassing the medical establishment and advertising miracle cures directly to the public. In the United States, the 1962 Kefauver-Harris Drug Amendments gave the Food and Drug Administration authority to regulate prescription drug advertisements in print and on TV and radio. The FDA insisted that all ads contain a summary of the drug's side effects, contraindications, warnings, and directions for use. An ad would also have to provide a "fair balance" of information about a drug's effectiveness, safety, and risks. These requirements proved too burdensome for a 30-second spot on TV or radio, so pharmaceutical companies focused on selling their drugs to physicians.

This practice changed in the early 1980s[4], when an enterprising, young marketer working for Boots Pharmaceuticals in Shreveport, LA decided to shift the paradigm and produce commercials to target consumers rather than doctors. On May 19, 1983, Boots aired the first broadcast television commercial in the United States for a prescription drug, the pain reliever Rufen. Within 48 hours, the FDA demanded that Boots discontinue the campaign, but the battle for DTC advertising was on.

In a 1985 policy statement, the FDA held fast to its 1962 position that any claims of a drug's efficacy had to be accurate and that ads must disclose side effects and other safety concerns. These requirements deterred DTC advertising for a decade before a campaign for the allergy medication *Claritin* changed the game. The *Claritin* ad never made any specific health claims; it merely presented images of a person breathing deeply and enjoying a sunny day outdoors, which was "*Claritin* clear." The ad never overtly stated what the medication was for but told viewers to ask their doctor about *Claritin*.

The *Claritin* ad posed a dilemma for the FDA. Could the agency require a drugmaker to list side effects to balance out claims

4 *https://www.statnews.com/2015/12/11/untold-story-tvs-first-prescription-drug-ad/*

of efficacy, if it made no claims of efficacy? That seemed to intrude on the advertiser's First Amendment rights. Thus, in 1997, the FDA relaxed its rules. The TV spots wouldn't have to contain all the downside information, as long as the ads referred viewers to print ads, toll-free phone numbers, or websites, where they could find the information, and urged people to talk to their doctors.

The door was open for the type of DTC drug advertisements that dominate the airwaves today. These ads practically instruct consumers to demand certain drugs from their prescribers. The result is problematic. Even if you believe, as I do, that the patient should make the ultimate decisions about their care, patients are not doctors. Armed with precious little information from a source with a clear financial interest, demanding patients can put a doctor in a terrible bind. Doctors who refuse the request because of concerns about the drug risk losing patients. On the other side of the coin, drug companies have been fined time and again for offering illegal compensation to healthcare providers who prescribe their drugs, often for "off-label" uses for which the drugs are not approved. It's not a good situation when doctors make medical decisions based on their own financial interests, rather than the patient's health. But the way we practice medicine today often puts practitioners in that dilemma.

DTC drug advertising has also opened up a huge revenue stream for TV and radio stations. Drug companies spent about \$360 million on DTC advertising in 1995, which swelled to \$1.3 billion in 1998, and surpassed \$5 billion in 2006. In 2021, Big Pharma spent an estimated \$8.1 billion on ads[5].

---

5 *Source: https://www.csrxp.org/big-pharma-watch-big-pharma-*

All of this money can't help but influence the TV networks and radio stations that have come to rely on the ad revenue. Are news programs more likely to ignore stories about dangerous drugs or the unethical practices of pharmaceutical companies? If so, where are the watchdogs who should protect the public? Who is telling the public that chronic dependence on various drugs is not the prescription for good health? Who is telling them that virtually all of these drugs would be unnecessary if they adopted a healthy lifestyle? Many of us in the wellness sector are trying to get this message out, but it is often lost in the saturation advertising that promises a new day courtesy of a pill. As a result, 97.5 percent of American healthcare spending goes toward treatment of manifested pathologies, while only 0.5 percent of that budget goes toward preventative care.

So, there you have some of the leading obstacles to an optimized healthspan. To overcome these impediments, we need a new *Tao* of bodily harmony that also supports emotional balance, mental clarity, and a peaceful, invigorated spirit. Believe me when I say that I know this need personally.

As my life story attests, I have at times been a workaholic. I studied rigorously for many years and then started a demanding career as a research professor. As my career expanded, I came to publish more than 400 peer-reviewed papers. I was put in charge of a 30-million-dollar building at a university and faced pressure to make good on the investment and the institution's faith in me. Along the way, I was lucky enough to marry a wonderful woman and have two lovely children. But

---

spent-8-1-billion-on-ads-pushing-high-priced-brand-name-prescription-drugs-in-2022/

even that did not put me at peace. Amid my daily workload, I was always searching, always yearning for the opportunity that would bring me back to my first, most earnest desire: to help people live their best lives.

This is perhaps why my study of NAD was such a personal as well as professional revelation. Here, perhaps, was the key to an optimized healthspan. And in helping others reach their fullest potential, I could find peace and unity in that pursuit. NAD would help me return to my uncarved block.

CHAPTER 5

ALL ROADS LEAD TO NAD

*"The Light of Inner Power radiates and heals.
Whosoever witnesses this healing is drawn to it.
Whosoever hears it looks to it in admiration."*

—Lao-Tzu, *Tao Te Ching*

As I studied age-related illness, I had to wonder, "Was NAD depletion the culprit?" The simple fact that lower levels of NAD coincided with age-related illness was not sufficient evidence, because, as scientists say, correlation is not causation. But before we get into the particulars of research and testing, I must provide a little background on what NAD actually is.

NAD, often abbreviated NAD+, stands for nicotinamide adenine dinucleotide, which is a coenzyme necessary for redox reactions. Let's break down that definition. An enzyme is a protein that acts as a catalyst in a biochemical reaction. The presence of an enzyme can speed up a reaction or enable the reaction to happen at a lower temperature or under less pressure. An enzyme enables the reaction but is not part of the reaction, in that it doesn't break down and contribute molecules to the new compound. A coenzyme is also an organic substance, but it's a non-protein molecule that an enzyme requires to perform its catalytic duty. Coenzymes are smaller molecules than enzymes and, importantly, do change their chemical structure during the catalytic reaction. This means that once NAD+ contributes to a chemical reaction, it's gone and must be replaced in order for the body to maintain its ability to produce energy.

Now, what is a redox reaction? You might be aware that the human body uses electrical charges for various functions, most notably for sending nerve impulses to and from the brain. On the cellular level, a redox reaction is a chemical process that involves the transfer of an electron from one molecule to another. On the full-body level, redox means we are using electricity to turn glucose into energy. This is why most sports drinks designed to replenish energy contain some type of glucose and electrolytes, which provide ions for electron transfer. From the importance of NAD+ in redox reactions, we can understand that NAD is essential for energy metabolism. This leads us to suspect that if we are sluggish, we might have insufficient NAD.

NAD+ is also an essential cofactor for non-redox processes. Again, this means it helps enzymes that couldn't do their jobs without it. These non-redox tasks cover several necessary cell functions, such as DNA repair, cell division, maintenance of metabolic pathways, gene expression, cellular senescence, the regulation of circadian rhythms, and immune response. If a body does not have sufficient levels of NAD+, all of these processes would suffer, and the body would become susceptible to frailty and diseases, such as cancer, as well as cognitive decline. None of this is good for lifespan or healthspan.

All told, NAD is essential to more than 500 biochemical reactions, which leads us to conclude that without NAD, there would be no life.

Over the past decade or more, many researchers had been assuming that suboptimal NAD was the culprit in a variety of maladies, such as chronic fatigue, chronic inflammation and pain, brain fog, and systemic illnesses, such as diabetes. But they lacked reliable evidence to prove their suspicions. They couldn't perform an in-depth study of NAD, because there was no reliable method available for measuring NAD levels. As a result, few physicians in the medical mainstream were paying any attention to developments in NAD research. Patients complaining of fatigue, inflammation, and other maladies were not screened for NAD deficiency, because doctors couldn't tell for certain they were deficient and wouldn't have known how to remedy NAD deficiency even if they found it.

The stumbling block was that testing of NAD levels relied on whole blood, so it was too costly and difficult to collect and process a sufficient number of samples. I recognized the necessity of developing an easy test for NAD levels, and after much trial and error, I designed the first successful test. In early 2019, we suspected we had a reliable test, and we further developed the process to work with a simple pinprick in 2020. The simplicity of this test allowed us to gather samples easily and even remotely.

However, even as we were gathering data through this testing, we had a problem. Nobody knew what the population profile was for NAD levels. Through our work with elderly, ill patients, we knew their range, and we assumed it was sub-optimal. But we didn't know what normal and optimal levels were for healthy, active people at other stages of life. We didn't know if NAD levels were naturally different in healthy men and women, or if different races charted differently. We assumed that NAD levels declined with age, but when approximately did the decline begin? What was the slope of the decline? Did external factors affect the slope of the decline?

Our research showed that NAD levels are highest in youngsters under twenty and decline with age, most sharply after age 30.

Then there was the question of optimizing NAD. What level should an individual shoot for? Is there a point where NAD levels become too high and we either see diminishing returns or negative effects? As a data-driven scientist, I wanted to collect as many samples as possible and screen for as many factors as possible. We needed to create a broad panel of biomarkers and cross-reference all samples according to age, sex, race, and physical condition so that we could do as deep a dive as possible. Almost four years after developing our test, we are still collecting and analyzing data. We shall continue to collect and analyze results, refining our processes as we go, to be able to make precise, targeted recommendations for our clients and improve our product offerings. What is the best way to optimize NAD levels?

Having determined that people could possibly regain their vitality through NAD optimization, we had to explore various methods and determine which were most efficacious. Here is where I feel obligated to warn anyone against methods that are costly and ineffective. Because of the promise of NAD optimization, many companies are offering supplements and processes they claim will raise NAD levels. But most NAD+ supplements simply do not work.

I don't say this as a producer of a competing line of products but as a biochemistry research scientist. When I began analyzing the performance of NAD+ supplements, my company was solely focused on biomarkers. In fact, *Jinfiniti* was established to test for longevity biomarkers. Biomarkers are measurable substances in the human body (or any organism), whose presence indicates a biological phenomenon, whether it be healthy homeostasis, some type of malady, or exposure to an environmental factor. We created panels to screen for essential biomarkers that indicate the likelihood of disease. Our goal was to identify issues far enough ahead of the onset of age-related disease, so a patient could make the necessary adjustments to prevent illness.

After we developed the NAD test, we had customers coming to us to find out their NAD levels. Many of these people had already tried different methods for raising their NAD levels. They wanted to know if they'd reached a level of optimization or if they could still do better. This testing led us to conclude that these patients had not been well served by the optimization methods they tried. So, it was only after this testing and some additional research that we determined that available supplements were not doing the job. Out of necessity, we decided to develop a more effective product. Why did the other supplements fall short? Allow me to explain.

First, many NAD supplements are made with the wrong molecule. Even though NAD+ is a coenzyme, it is still a large molecule. In fact, it is too large to pass what we call "the gut barrier."

This is the intestinal membrane that functions as a bodily defense by restricting the passage of ions, molecules, and cells from the gut into the bloodstream. These "whole NAD" supplements mostly pass through your intestinal tract into your toilet, optimizing little more than your stool.

Unfortunately, companies that make this kind of "rookie mistake" can't be expected to get much else right. They source their products with less fresh or lower-quality ingredients. They also can't confirm the efficacy of their products, because they don't perform any in-house testing. They don't analyze their customers' NAD levels before and after using their products, so they have no way of demonstrating that their products actually raised their customers' NAD levels. Also, because these companies do not test, they don't know what dosage of their product to recommend.

In my laboratory, we have tested some of the biggest brands in the world, which spend millions of dollars advertising their ineffective products. We also have clients come to us after using some of these supplements, often for extended periods of time at great expense. We've found these clients have only experienced an incremental improvement of maybe 20-40 percent at best. By contrast, we have helped clients gain 300 percent increases in only four weeks.

Why NAD IVs Don't Work

One method of NAD+ enhancement that's been around for decades is intravenous infusion. This consists of an intravenous drip of a solution containing NAD+ molecules. Patients can receive this treatment in a healthcare provider's office. It usually takes a few hours and might be repeated several times over a span of a week or more. This therapy has been used for neurological conditions, such as Parkinson's disease, or for infectious diseases, such as Lyme disease and post-COVID syndrome. In both situations, truly effective and reliable remedies have proven elusive. IV infusion has also been used to boost energy and as an anti-aging treatment. As you can imagine, this treatment is expensive and time-consuming, and for these reasons, patients easily get the impression that this is the Gold Standard of NAD+ optimization. However, the results we have observed do not live up to the hype.

First, we must note there are a number of limitations to this treatment. Many patients report uncomfortable, even painful, side effects. Its efficacy is questionable and even the best outcomes seem to be temporary. The inconvenience and expense of uncertain outcomes should give any patient pause.

My first question in approaching any treatment is, "Where's the science?" To my knowledge, which is by no means casual, no peer-reviewed study has ever been published supporting this practice. Of course, there is no shortage of anecdotal evidence, which seems equally balanced pro and con. It appears from my review of various accounts of patient outcomes that IV infusion of NAD+ can be effective for neurological conditions, including Parkinson's, Alzheimer's, and Lyme's diseases, as well as for addictions. The absence of reliable remedies for these conditions weighs in favor of trying IV infusion for relief of symptoms. Unfortunately, even when the therapy seems to work on these conditions, the benefits are only temporary.

Individuals who desire NAD+ enhancement for anti-aging purposes or to improve physical performance do not seem to benefit, even in the short term, from IV infusion.

Because we are trying to improve health and functionality on the cellular level, the most basic and important question might be, "Does IV infusion increase intracellular NAD+?" Since there is no published research to review, we conducted our own study of 10 healthy individuals. We measured their NAD before and after five infusion sessions over 10 days. We found that the baseline NAD+ levels inside their cells were not elevated, let alone optimized. There was simply no evidence of an increase. However, our study did not end there. We provided these same subjects with our formulation of NAD precursors, which we shall discuss later, and their intracellular NAD+ levels increased significantly. Nine of the 10 subjects quickly reached a level of NAD optimization.

Remember what we said about supplements made from whole NAD+? The molecule is too large to pass through the gut barrier. Then how should we expect anything different from whole NAD+ in the bloodstream? The molecules are also too large to pass through the vacuoles of the cell membranes to enter the cells and reach the mitochondria where they are needed.

Anyone considering NAD+ IV infusion must also be wary of side effects. In our study of this issue, we noted a significant increase of the inflammation biomarker hs-CRP in 70 percent of the test subjects. By significant, I mean a 3-to-10-fold increase. We might expect this outcome after surgery or a serious infection that jolts the body's immune system into overdrive. Apparently, the body reads the influx of NAD+ as some kind of invasion. The liver, our major organ for detoxifying our system, treats the infused NAD as a foreign substance it must flush out. This side effect suggests that IV infusion creates the risk of shock to the body, and we certainly wouldn't recommend this method when other viable processes exist.

To summarize, our findings on IV infusion revealed four key points:

- NAD+ IV therapy may benefit individuals suffering from neurological disorders and infectious diseases.
- NAD+ IV therapy is not efficacious for anti-aging therapy or to attain performance goals.
- Health benefits from NAD+ intravenous infusion are temporary and therefore may not be worth the risk, inconvenience, and expense.
- Since safer, more effective, more affordable, and more convenient methods of NAD+ enhancement exist, we cannot recommend IV infusion.

Does a Subcutaneous Injection of NAD+ Elevate Levels?

A subcutaneous injection (SubQ or SQ) is the use of a medical syringe to inject medication below the skin into fatty tissue. From there the medicine enters the bloodstream. Diabetics use SQ for insulin, but SQ can also be used for blood thinners, birth control, or any medication where you want a timed release into the patient's system. Pumps and patches operate under the same principle.

We have found that SubQ of NAD+ can modestly elevate NAD levels but rarely achieves optimum levels for maximum benefits.

The efficacy of SQ certainly depends on the dosage and frequency of injections. It is advised that SubQ users of NAD+ check their NAD levels to determine whether their protocol is working for them. Due to the high cost, invasive nature of injections, and insufficient efficacy for SubQ NAD+, we strongly recommend using oral NAD precursors to optimize NAD levels.

If Whole NAD+ Does Not Work Via Supplements or IV Infusion, How Can We Optimize NAD+?

Imagine that you are a music lover and would love to have a baby grand piano as the centerpiece of your living room. You measure your front door and then go to the piano store. But none of the models will fit through your entryway. Should you give up your dream of that beautiful Steinway? Of course not! Ask any piano salesman, and he'll tell you they can remove the legs from the piano and easily get it through your door, and then they will reassemble it inside your home. So, why can't we do this with NAD?

What I am suggesting is that we take smaller molecules which are the building blocks of NAD and supplement them. Then, once inside the cell, these molecules will come together to form the larger NAD molecules which would not have made it past the gut barrier or fit through the cell's vacuoles. These building blocks are called precursors because they come before the NAD itself. As I considered different approaches to NAD supplementation, I knew the only effective method must be based on precursor molecules.

My goal was to create a supplement in water-soluble, powder form, which, in addition to being effective, would have a pleasant taste. I wanted to stay away from capsules because they require extra ingredients that don't deliver any benefit. I wanted it to taste good so people wouldn't dread taking it, and because I worried about the compound breaking down in the digestive tract. If it had a pleasant taste, people could hold it in their mouths, swishing it around, for maybe a minute, and much could be absorbed sublingually for better effect. That couldn't happen with a capsule.

So then, what precursors would suit our purposes? An important consideration for efficacy was that the precursors we chose should take the least amount of energy to convert to NAD. Of all the possibilities, two strong contenders stood out: NMN and NR.

Let's start with the first of these, nicotinamide mononucleotide, or NMN. You can tell by the name that it has some of the component atoms of nicotinamide adenine dinucleotide, or NAD. I knew that NMN would be a reliable NAD precursor since it is so closely related chemically and would need very little energy for synthesis. But I also knew there had been problems with NMN supplements, including headaches and sleepiness. I needed to balance the NMN with other ingredients that would relieve those side effects and contribute to our ultimate goal of forming NAD within human cells.

As for NR, or nicotinamide riboside, it's a form of vitamin B3 that can be converted into NAD through a simple, two-step enzymatic process. NR supplementation has shown promise in increasing NAD levels in various preclinical and clinical studies, making it another potentially valuable precursor. Now, some readers might see B3 mentioned and think immediately of the B vitamin that causes the famous "niacin flush." This nutrient is recognized as beneficial for regulating cholesterol and blood pressure, boosting brain function, and improving skin. Most people tolerate supplements in low doses. Unfortunately, supplementing at the level necessary to meaningfully affect NAD levels can lead to health concerns. So, let us digress momentarily to explain the situation with niacin.

The Niacin Fallacy: How Supplementing This B Vitamin Can Cause Additional Health Problems

Of course, I was not the only one experimenting with NAD+ precursors. Some studies focused on nicotinic acid (NA), popularly known as niacin, or Vitamin B3. One such study, entitled, *Niacin Cures Systemic NAD+ Deficiency and Improves Muscle Performance in Adult-Onset Mitochondrial Myopathy* was published in the journal *Cell Metabolism*, Volume 32, Issue 1, 7 July 2020. This study claimed to show that niacin improves muscle strength and symptoms of fatty liver in mitochondrial myopathy patients, and that niacin boosts muscle mitochondrial biogenesis and respiratory chain activity in humans. This is all very positive. However, when we examined niacin (NA), we found it was not a particularly effective NAD precursor, and supplementing Niacin in large does could raise health concerns. Niacin does not significantly increase NAD levels in most people, but we have found extremely high and potentially harmful levels of NAD (>150μM) in a few individuals using high doses of niacin (500-2000mg daily). This finding led us to warn heavy niacin users that they should measure their NAD levels using our NAD test to find out whether their NAD levels are too low or too high.

Here's a story from a *Jinfiniti* client (a respected medical professional) who had tried to optimize NAD with heavy doses of niacin:

For over two decades, I struggled with intractable insomnia—an affliction that robbed me of restful nights and, undoubtedly, shortened my healthspan. I tried everything: prescription medications, lifestyle changes, specialized therapies, and countless supplements. Nothing worked. Other medical professionals and sleep specialists had no real answers for me. I spent thousands of dollars and many years- not to mention countless sleepless nights- searching for a solution, but I remained trapped in a cycle of exhaustion.

As a physician specializing in functional and anti-aging medicine, I understood the critical role that sleep plays in longevity. Without deep, restorative sleep, the body cannot properly repair itself, cognitive function declines, and the risk of chronic disease skyrockets. My insomnia wasn't just an inconvenience—it was a direct threat to my long-term health.

At the same time, I had been taking high doses of niacin for years—2000 mg per day—to help control my lipid levels and blood pressure. Niacin is a powerful vasodilator and a well-known strategy for cardiovascular health. It worked beautifully for me. My cholesterol levels were optimal, and my blood pressure remained in a safe range. I had no reason to question it—until I took Dr. Jin-Xiong She's Intracellular NAD test.

The results were shocking. My NAD levels were 50% higher than the highest end of the optimal range.

This revelation stopped me in my tracks. NAD is a crucial coenzyme responsible for mitochondrial energy production, DNA repair, and cellular resilience. It's widely regarded as a cornerstone of anti-aging medicine. The entire longevity field emphasizes increasing NAD levels as we age. But in my case, I had inadvertently driven my NAD too high—far beyond what was beneficial.

At that moment, I didn't even know what the potential harm could be. But with Dr. She's guidance, I was about to find out.

The Experiment: Lowering My NAD

Determined to restore balance, I decided to lower my niacin intake to bring my NAD levels down. I gradually tapered my daily dose, cutting it down significantly, per Dr. She's suggestion. My NAD levels did drop, but they still hovered near the upper limits of the optimal range.

Then something remarkable happened.

As my NAD levels declined, my sleep began to improve. For the first time in over 20 years, I was sleeping through the night. The transformation was astounding. I felt more refreshed, more energized, and—ironically—more alive than I had in years.

But there was a trade-off. Without niacin, my lipids worsened, and my blood pressure crept up. I had to make a difficult decision: continue taking niacin to manage my cardiovascular health or eliminate it completely to maintain my newfound ability to sleep.

I chose to stop niacin altogether.

At first, I was concerned about my lipid and blood pressure numbers, but those were issues I could address with other interventions. What mattered most was that my insomnia—the condition that had plagued me for two decades—was gone. Completely gone.

What stunned me the most was that no one in the medical or longevity community had ever made this connection before. We hear endlessly about the benefits of NAD and how we should optimize it, but no one talks about the potential risks of having levels that are too high.

Yet, here I was—a physician who had spent years in the anti-aging field—discovering first-hand that excess NAD could be a hidden driver of insomnia.

This is why testing is so crucial. If I had never taken Dr. She's Intracellular NAD test or followed his personalized guidance, I would have never uncovered this connection. I would still be taking niacin, still suffering from relentless insomnia, and still searching for answers in all the wrong places.

It's time for a paradigm shift in how we think about NAD optimization. While most people do need to increase their NAD levels as they age, some—like me—are unknowingly pushing them too high, creating unintended consequences. As with all supplements, it's not a one-size-fits-all situation. Different people respond differently to the very same supplement.

Especially in this case, if you're taking niacin or an NAD precursor, you must test. You're flying blind if you don't.

As we say in medicine: **the dose makes the poison**.

This doctor makes important observations about dosage levels and the necessity of precision testing to understand what exactly your course of supplementation is doing inside your body. We shall return to this discussion a little later. But we should note that in addition to the insomnia our doctor friend complained of, niacin overdose can produce numerous disconcerting symptoms. According to the Mayo Clinic, these include:

- Severe skin flushing combined with dizziness
- Rapid heartbeat
- Itching
- Nausea and vomiting
- Abdominal pain
- Diarrhea
- Gout
- Rash

Niacin has also been linked to liver damage and strokes, so most healthcare professionals will only recommend it for cholesterol regulation when a patient can't take statins. These symptoms raise concerns about the prudence of supplementing large doses of niacin to raise NAD levels.

Clinical trials have shown that nicotinamide (NAM) can modestly increase NAD levels in some individuals. However, it does not increase NAD levels at all in many users and only increases NAD to optimum levels in a tiny fraction of individuals tested. Ultimately, we rejected NAM and NA for our supplement formula in favor of more effective and safer precursors.

Our observations showed that both NMN and NR were effective precursors. The question became, "Which one to choose?" As it turns out, we needed both. Rather than being competitors, NMN and NR complement each other in the NAD biosynthesis pathway. NMN takes a more direct route, but NR serves as an indirect source by first being converted to NMN. Anyone who has ever lost power due to a storm is happy to have an auxiliary generator, and this is precisely the role that

NR plays. It's also possible that different tissues and organs (as well as different microbiomes) might prefer one precursor over the other. This redundancy enables the body to adapt to varying conditions and ensures a steady supply of fresh NAD. Of course, we didn't know this at the time, and we had to go through countless rounds of testing. (As mentioned earlier, NR (nicotinamide riboside) is closely related to NA (niacin), since they are both forms of vitamin B3. But NR did not cause the concerns that accompany high doses of niacin.)

My wife and I set up a laboratory in our kitchen. My wife has a PhD in biochemistry, so she became the chief cook, selecting and mixing ingredients. Working nights and weekends for well over a year, we must have tested a couple thousand combinations of compounds in various proportions. Since my wife was the cook, I was the chief taster. If I tried it and didn't die, then she would take it. Interestingly, we found that the best proportion of ingredients expressed the Golden Ratio. Mathematicians have studied this relationship since antiquity. You may have seen the ratio expressed as the Fibonacci Spiral or the Golden Spiral, which looks like a perfect snail shell. In this way, we discovered that our NAD experimentation not only harkens back to the *Tao* of Lao-Tzu, but it also bears some relation to the elegant mathematics of Pythagoras, Euclid, and Fibonacci. We took this as a very good omen and were not surprised at all when some researchers started calling NAD "the golden nucleotide."

CHAPTER 6

THE DIFFERENCE BETWEEN HEALTHSPAN AND LIFESPAN

"Is fame worth the sacrifice of our true nature? Does wealth compensate for the loss of ourselves? Which causes more suffering—accumulating things or letting them all go?"

—Lao-Tzu, *Tao Te Ching*

It is a generally accepted maxim that there is no greater wealth than a long life. But what if that life is spent in needless suffering? The Irish satirist Jonathan Swift presented this paradox in his celebrated novel, *Gulliver's Travels*. On one of his voyages, Gulliver reaches the island of Luggnagg, where he encounters the struldbrugs, a race of people who are immortal. Unfortunately, they do not have the gift of eternal youth, so they suffer the infirmities of old age without end. They are so incapacitated after the age of eighty that the law considers them legally dead. A particularly poignant scene has Gulliver witnessing the bedridden, unconscious existence of an ancient struldbrug. In this moment, we see how useless an endless lifespan would be without the health and vitality to enjoy those added years. Yet, one might argue that this is the type of existence that modern medicine is producing.

Before we get too deeply into this discussion, allow me to define some terms. When we talk about the lifespan of a species, we're referring to the maximum potential length of life, which for humans presently is about 120 years. Life expectancy, on the other hand, is how long the average person in a certain place at a certain time is likely to live. Eventually, we will address healthspan, which is the maximum term of years for healthy, active living.

According to the U.S. Census Bureau[6], the average life expectancy for the total population in the United States increased by almost 10 years from 69.7 years in 1960 to 79.4 years in 2015. In 1960, a person retiring at age 65 would on average enjoy only five years of retirement. In 2015, that 65-year-old could reasonably expect 15 years. The Bureau attributes the lengthier lifespans to a combination of factors, including "increases in vaccinations, continued decreases in infectious diseases and cardiovascular mortality, and the effectiveness of prevention programs related to smoking, alcohol consumption, and promotion of physical activity." A longer life, free of labor, is certainly desirable. But just how golden might we expect those added years to be?

In 1980, the life expectancy in the United States was in a statistical dead heat with other large, prosperous nations. Life expectancy in the United States was 73.7 years, while the average of the "comparable countries" was 74.5 years. However,

6 *https://www.census.gov/content/dam/Census/library/publications/2020/demo/p25-1145.pdf*

as life expectancy has continued to increase over the ensuing decades, the United States has started to fall behind. In 2019, before the COVID outbreak, U.S. life expectancy was 78.8 years, while life expectancy in comparable countries was at 82.6 years. The United States lagged behind despite spending almost twice as much per capita on medical treatment: the U.S. average was $12,197 in 2021, as opposed to the average healthcare spend of $6,345 in comparable countries. What does the vastly higher healthcare expenditure say about the quality of life for U.S. citizens?

According to several studies, Americans today are living longer but enjoying fewer healthy years. In 2001, Eileen M. Crimmins, a professor of gerontology at the University of Southern California published her findings on the increases in age-related diseases in both men and women aged 70 or older, observed from 1984 to 1995. These conditions include arthritis, diabetes, cancer, hypertension, stroke, and heart disease.

In 2011,[7] Dr, Crimmins and USC postdoctoral fellow Hiram Beltrán-Sánchez revisited this problem. Their analysis of available data found that an extended lifespan also meant an increase in the number of years living with morbidity:

> *The analysis showed that a man who was 20 years old in 1998 could expect to live about 55 additional years, spending about 10 of those years with serious disease and 3.8 with limited mobility. In contrast, a man who was 20 years old in 2006 could expect to live longer still (56.1 additional years) but spend more time with disease (12.3 years) and lack of mobility (5.8 years). Women's average life spans, although still about 5 years longer than those*

7 *https://www.ncbi.nlm.nih.gov/pmc/articles/PMC3060013*

of men, increased at a slower rate than men's, while their years of morbidity increased at a higher rate.

Crimmins noted, "We do not appear to be moving to a world where we die without experiencing disease, functioning loss, and disability."

Findings like these convinced the World Health Organization[8] to begin thinking about life expectancy differently. Length was not a clear enough indicator of quality. Thus, WHO adopted a metric called Health-adjusted life expectancy (HALE or HLE), which is the average number of years a person can expect to live in full health, unencumbered by debilitating illnesses or injuries. WHO began compiling HALE data in 1999. According to WHO[9], a 60-year-old male in the United States in 2019 can expect 15.59 years of a healthy lifespan, while a woman the same age can expect 17.06 years. In various settings, HALE seems to lag about five years behind life expectancy, meaning the average person can expect five years of disability due to illness or injury towards the end of life.

But does HALE tell the whole story? How much of the "slowing down" that occurs with age does HALE fail to account for? What about the symptoms that encumber individuals, but fall short of a disease diagnosis? Aches, pains, inflexibility, inflammation, memory lapses. The vast majority of older adults will deal with these symptoms. Their complaints will not rise to

8 *https://www.verywellhealth.com/understanding-healthy-life-expectancy-2223919*

9 *https://www.who.int/data/gho/data/indicators/indicator-details/GHO/gho-ghe-hale-healthy-life-expectancy-at-birth*

the level of a disability but will certainly diminish their quality of life.

Which brings us to the next point. How many older adults are taking medications to deal with symptoms associated with old age? And is the practice of prescribing such drugs trending earlier and earlier in life as a precaution? And, importantly, do the drugs taken to alleviate a specific symptom cause side effects which wear away at the patient's overall health and quality of life? Considering the amount of money Americans spend on prescription drugs, these are questions worth asking.

The most prescribed medications for seniors in the United States are used to treat high blood pressure, type II diabetes, high cholesterol, coronary artery disease, and acid reflux. Yet many people can avoid these conditions by making healthy lifestyle choices. Unfortunately, too many individuals delay making changes in their lifestyle until the onset of disease. By this time, it's difficult to manage or reverse a condition without medication. The goal should be to get the patient healthy enough to discontinue the prescription. However, too few healthcare providers think in these terms, so once they put a patient on a drug that seems to alleviate symptoms, it's as if the prescription has been carved in stone. The next symptom will be met with another drug, and on and on.

I am not the only researcher who believes that there is an excessive medication problem among the elderly in the United States. Writing for *Adviser Magazine*[10], Dr. Robert Drapkin, MD, FACP notes that, "As people age, the likelihood of being

10 *https://www.lifehealth.com/american-are-living-longer-but-not-always-healthier/*

prescribed more than one medication rises. Individuals aged 65 to 69 take an average of 15 prescriptions per year, while those from 80 to 84 take an average of 18." That's an astounding number of pills, especially when we consider that "15 to 25 percent of drugs used by seniors is considered unnecessary or inappropriate and the economic impact of medication-related problems is estimated at $177.4 billion per year, rivaling that of Alzheimer's disease, cancer, diabetes, and cardiovascular disease."

Dr. Drapkin paints a picture of vulnerable seniors despoiling their life savings to pay for the next batch of ineffectual pharmaceuticals. He cites "75 percent of Medicare-eligible households" spending "at least $10,000 on healthcare during their last five years of life," with the average outlay totaling $38,688. For most American seniors, as well as for the federal Medicare budget, this level of spending is unsustainable. Worse yet, these seniors aren't buying mild medicinals, which might not work, but at least will cause no harm. Dr. Drapkin tells us, "*The Journal of General Internal Medicine* found that doctors in the U.S. routinely prescribe potentially harmful drugs to older patients. Many commonly prescribed drugs can do more harm than good, because they remain in elderly patients' systems longer, causing higher rates of complications."

A heavy reliance on prescription medication also raises the risk of a dangerous interaction among the drugs. Drug interactions in the elderly[11] significantly increase the risk of:

- Falls and fractures

11 *https://www.webmd.com/healthy-aging/common-medications-for-older-adults*

- Dehydration
- Difficulty performing daily tasks
- Cognitive difficulties, memory lapses, and brain fog
- Confusion and decreased awareness of surroundings
- Nutrient deficiencies

Many adverse interactions are known, so the drugs carry warnings. Unfortunately, prescribers and patients often miss the warnings. The result is a heightened risk of hospitalization and death.

We must also note the problem of compliance in older adults. For a prescription to work, it must be taken regularly at the appropriate dosage. When seniors are taking a dozen pills a day or more, it's easy to become confused about which pill to take when, or how often. Mistakes undermine the effectiveness of the drug, so patients wind up spending a lot of money for little to no benefit, while still risking side effects and harmful interactions.

Another danger to older adults comes from their diminished ability to recover from injuries. Falls are especially dangerous for seniors whose balance and reflexes decline with age. On its website, The National Safety Council[12] notes:

> *As our population ages, the prevalence of falls among older adults is increasing. According to the Centers for Disease Control and Prevention (CDC), more than one in four older adults report a fall each year. In 2021, 38,742 older adults aged 65 and older*

12 *https://injuryfacts.nsc.org/home-and-community/safety-topics/older-adult-falls/*

died from preventable falls, and nearly 2.9 million were treated in emergency departments. Over the past 10 years, older adult fall deaths have increased by 60 percent, while emergency department visits have increased 20 percent. At the same time, the number of fall deaths among individuals younger than 65 increased 23 percent, but emergency department visits have decreased 37 percent.

From personal observation, I understand how devastating a fall can be for an older person. My father-in-law suffered a fall in his 70s and was never the same. This is all too common an occurrence among the elderly, who do not heal as fast or as thoroughly as younger people. Sadly, studies have shown that about 50 percent of people over 65 who fall and break a hip die within six months.

The NSC also warns that seniors are vulnerable to a range of potentially deadly, accidental injuries, such as:

- **FIRES** — Seniors are 3.5 times more likely to die in fires than the general population, accounting for roughly 930 deaths per year. The clothing fire death rate is 14 times higher than the rate for people under 65.
- **DROWNING** — About 300 older adults die by drowning annually, mostly associated in pools, bathtubs, and spas.
- **TRANSPORTATION** — More than 200 older adults die each year from crashes involving off-highway vehicles, bicycles, and e-scooters.
- **CARBON MONOXIDE POISONING** — About 45 older consumers die each year from CO poisoning produced by heating devices, generators, and other engine-driven tools.

- **BED RAIL ENTRAPMENT** — Safety devices meant to protect seniors from falling out of bed have been linked to about 16 deaths per year. Entrapment often results in suffocation.

Even when injuries from these accidents are not fatal, victims can suffer prolonged, excruciating pain and disability. How tragic that a preventable accident can rob an older person of health and mobility, making their final years a grim footnote to an otherwise active and joyous life. How sad that so many individuals who have reaped "bonus years" from increased life expectancy, spend that extra time in nursing facilities and assisted living because they can no longer care for themselves.

We have not quite reached the state of Swift's struldbrugs, but the trend in modern medicine is to prolong life by alleviating symptoms, but without restoring the vitality that makes life worth living. Western medicine exists under a cloud of inevitability, bordering on defeatism. It is the sense that age-related decline must come, so we can only make older patients comfortable until their systems fail. This palliative approach might ultimately be necessary since we cannot live forever. But my research strongly suggests that we are throwing in the towel too soon. Restoring and maintaining vitality is possible through a comprehensive approach that includes NAD optimization.

Therefore, if the human lifespan is 120 years, why should life expectancy in prosperous nations be roughly 80 years old? Why are we only living for two-thirds of our potential? And why should health-adjusted life expectancy be even less? My research strongly suggests that NAD can be the key to achieving optimal lifespan and healthspan. It is time to use that key to unlock the possibilities.

CHAPTER 7

THE BASICS OF NAD

"Abundant Inner Power is like an infant. ...
All day the infant may cry, but is never hoarse.
Its harmony is perfect."

—Lao-Tzu, *Tao Te Ching*

Systemic health depends on organ health; organ health depends on tissue health; tissue health depends on cellular health. But if healthy cells are the building blocks for a healthy human, we have to ask ourselves, "What makes for healthy cells?" As a microbiologist, I have studied cell composition, and I understand how molecules act as micronutrients to aid cell function. I can say without fear of contradiction that when it comes to helping our cells function optimally, no other molecule comes close to NAD.

Time and again, I have seen how optimizing levels of NAD leads to a decrease in pain, inflammation, fatigue, and brain fog, as mental clarity, stamina, energy, muscle recovery, and youthful vigor all increase. Clients have reported brighter moods, better sleep, higher libido, and more satisfying sexual relations after achieving NAD optimization. These improvements suggest that we have discovered a powerful "bio-hack" with enormous potential for rolling back the problems of aging to allow our clients to enjoy peak performance once again.

But to understand how NAD+ works within a cell, we must first refresh our understanding of human cells. So, allow me to review the basics.

A cell is the smallest organic unit that performs all of life's processes. These include:

- **STRUCTURE AND SUPPORT** — Cells are the basic building blocks of an organism. Within each cell, there is a coded program that instructs the cell to participate in the formation of a discrete part of the body: organ, bone, blood, muscle, etc. But cells also have their own structural support: a permeable membrane that defines the limits of the cell.
- **GROWTH** — Complex organisms, such as humans, grow by multiplying cells. Cells multiply by dividing in two via a process called mitosis.
- **TRANSPORT** — Cells import nutrients and expel waste.
- **ENERGY PRODUCTION** — Cells turn nutrients into energy.
- **METABOLISM** — Cells perform chemical reactions that enable various biological processes.
- **REPRODUCTION** — Humans reproduce when a single cell from a male, the sperm, penetrates a single cell from a female, the ovum, resulting in fertilization. From there, mitosis takes over, and a child forms in the womb.

Human cells are differentiated into various types and subtypes. In reviewing these, you will note the frequent use of the suffix "cyte," which refers to a cell. The major cells of the human body include:

- **RED BLOOD CELLS** — The most common cell in the body, erythrocytes transport oxygen, carbon dioxide, nutrients, and other substances throughout the body.
- **WHITE BLOOD CELLS** — Essential to the immune system, white blood cells fight against infection, inflammation, and other diseases. Platelets are a type of WBC instrumental in blood clotting.
- **SKIN CELLS** — Your skin is your largest organ and is composed mainly of keratinocytes, which form the protective layer of the epidermis, and melanocytes, which produce pigment and protect us from ultraviolet radiation (e.g., sunlight). We also have Langerhans cells, which help fight infection, and Merkel cells that support our sense of touch.
- **MYOCYTES** — These are the cells that make up our muscular system. Cardiomyocytes are specialized muscle cells that keep the heart pumping.
- **STEM CELLS** — Undifferentiated cells found in bone marrow can morph into other types of cells.
- **BONE CELLS** — Classified as osteoclasts, osteoblasts, and osteocytes, different types of bone cells serve different functions.
- **CHONDROCYTES** — Consisting mostly of collagen and proteoglycans, these cells are found in cartilage.
- **NEURONS** — Nerve cells enable communication between different parts of your body and your brain. These

cells can carry messages from your brain to other parts of your body via electrical impulses.

- **FAT CELLS** — The human body has white adipocytes, which store energy as triglycerides, and brown adipocytes, which burn energy as heat. As we age, we produce fewer white fat cells and more brown fat cells.
- **SEX CELLS** — Also called gametes, these are the ovum in the female and the sperm in the male.

Although the different types of cells have distinctive characteristics, they have a similar composition, consisting of these parts:

- **CELL MEMBRANE** — Every cell is enclosed within a membrane which holds the inside in and keeps the outside out. The membrane upholds the integrity of the cell, acting as the gatekeeper for materials trying to enter through openings called vacuoles.
- **NUCLEUS** — The control center of the cell is a fluid nucleoplasm enclosed in a nuclear membrane. The nucleus contains threads of chromatin which contain deoxyribonucleic acid (DNA), the genetic material of the cell. Also within the nucleus is a dense region of ribonucleic acid (RNA), which is the site of ribosome formation. Ribosomes form proteins from amino acids.
- **CYTOPLASM** — This gel-like fluid is the medium for chemical reactions within the cell.
- **ORGANELLES** — Swimming in the pool of cytoplasm are tiny "organs" of various types that perform specific functions.

How cells operate is infinitely fascinating. On a microscopic scale, they are worlds unto themselves. They are as mysterious as the deepest oceans. Science is only beginning to understand how and why they function as they do. But we do know that a variety of functions are essential for life and that NAD assists in virtually all of them. Here is a brief list of the powerful benefits we have determined NAD delivers:

- **TELOMERE SHORTENING** — Telomeres are the protective caps at the end of our chromosomes, the threadlike structures that contain our DNA. The gradual shortening of telomeres over time is a hallmark of the aging process. As telomeres shorten, cells may lose their ability to divide and function properly. NAD+ plays a crucial role in cell division and other functions by supporting the activity of enzymes called sirtuins, which are involved in DNA repair and maintenance. Sirtuins require NAD+ as a coenzyme to function effectively, so a decline in levels of NAD+ can impair the sirtuins' ability to promote telomere stability and repair. In other words, as NAD+ levels decline with age, enzymes that depend on NAD+ can't do their jobs as well.
- **DEREGULATED NUTRIENT SENSING** — Cells need fuel to function. Nutrient sensing is the process that allows the cell to recognize and respond to fuel substrates, such as glucose. NAD+ serves as a critical cofactor of enzymes such as sirtuins, which are the key regulators of nutrient sensing pathways. When nutrient sensing becomes disrupted, often due to poor diet and a sedentary lifestyle, what follows is metabolic dysfunction and age-related diseases, including diabetes. Replenishing NAD+ levels will support sirtuin activity and restore balance in nutrient sensing.

- **STEM CELL EXHAUSTION** — Stem cells are essential for the regeneration and repair of various tissues, but their capacity to divide and differentiate declines with age. When NAD+ levels are low, sirtuin activity drops off, leading to inefficient DNA repair and genomic instability within stem cells, which in turn accelerates stem cell exhaustion and compromises tissue repair. By bolstering NAD levels, it's possible to enhance sirtuin function and potentially rejuvenate stem cell activity.
- **DISABLED MICROAUTOPHAGY** — Microautophagy is a cellular process responsible for degrading and recycling damaged organelles and proteins through direct engulfment by lysosomes. Autophagy literally means "self-eating" or "self-devouring," and refers to the consumption of worn-out cell components. In other words, it's how cells clean house. Again, sirtuins are intricately involved in maintaining cellular quality control mechanisms, including autophagy, which are essential to overall health. When NAD+ levels decline, sirtuin activity may be compromised, impacting microautophagy and other autophagic processes. This can result in the accumulation of cellular debris and impaired organelle quality. In essence, the cells become cluttered with poorly functioning components that ought to be replaced. This disarray will ultimately contribute to cellular dysfunction and aging.
- **INFLAMMAGING** — This term, which looks like a typo, refers to an age-related increase in the levels of pro-inflammatory markers in blood and tissues. Inflammaging is considered a strong risk factor for numerous diseases that are highly prevalent in elderly individuals and frequently cause disability. This chronic, low-grade inflammation is closely intertwined with NAD levels, because,

yet again, sirtuins, which regulate inflammation and immune responses, rely on NAD to get the job done. As NAD levels naturally decline with age, sirtuin activity may decrease, leading to a state of chronic inflammation, which can accompany a range of age-related conditions, including neurodegenerative diseases, cardiovascular issues, and metabolic disorders. By replenishing NAD levels, we can promote healthier aging and reduce the risk of various age-related diseases.

- **MITOCHONDRIAL DYSFUNCTION** — Mitochondria are the powerhouse of our cells, responsible for generating adenosine triphosphate (ATP), the cellular energy currency. NAD plays a critical role as a coenzyme in the electron transport chain, a fundamental process in mitochondrial ATP synthesis. However, as NAD levels decline with age, the efficiency of mitochondrial function may deteriorate, leading to impaired energy production and an increase in oxidative stress. (There's a great deal to be said about the role of oxidative stress in cellular health. Sufficient for now is to understand that cells contain free radicals, i.e., oxygen-containing molecules with an uneven number of electrons, which react easily with other molecules. We call this process oxidation, and it can be beneficial or harmful, depending on the molecules involved. A healthy diet contains plenty of antioxidants, e.g., vitamins A, C, and E, to prevent detrimental oxidation.) By maintaining optimal NAD levels, it's possible to support the function of key enzymes involved in mitochondrial energy production, potentially mitigating mitochondrial dysfunction, reducing harmful oxidation, and promoting cellular vitality.
- **CELLULAR SENESCENCE** — Cellular senescence is a state where cells lose their ability to divide and function

properly, often as a response to various stressors or DNA damage contributing to aging-related diseases and tissue dysfunction. Sirtuins play a crucial role in regulating and controlling the process of senescence, and as we've frequently noted, sirtuins need NAD to perform. Thus, the age-related decline of NAD levels can promote the accumulation of senescent cells in tissues. These senescent cells are often called zombie cells, because they stop working, but continue to secrete inflammatory and tissue-degrading molecules. They are The Walking Dead of our cellular ecosystem. Researchers have found[13] that higher levels of specific senescent biomarkers, such as GDF15, VEGFA, PARC, and MMP2, are associated with an increased risk of death. Some of these biomarkers also indicate a higher likelihood of chronic diseases, such as heart disease and certain types of cancers.

- **LOSS OF PROTEOSTASIS** — Protein homeostasis or 'proteostasis' is the process that regulates proteins within the cell to maintain good health. Cells convert proteins to energy through highly complex, interconnected pathways of synthesis and degradation. As some cell components are affected, others adjust to restore balance. Cellular health depends on the components that put the 'stasis' in proteostasis. When one or more of these proteostasis influencers are disrupted, improperly folded or misfolded proteins lead to protein aggregation[14]. This buildup of improperly processed cellular protein leads to a wide range of pathologies, including Alzheimer's disease, Parkinson's disease, amyotrophic lateral sclerosis

13 *https://discoverysedge.mayo.edu/2023/11/16/health-and-zombie-cells-in-aging/*

14 *https://pubmed.ncbi.nlm.nih.gov/11831622/*

(ALS or Lou Gehrig's disease), Huntington's disease, dementia with Lewy bodies, frontotemporal diseases, and multiple system atrophy. NAD is essential for proteostasis activity. Therefore, by replenishing NAD levels, it may be possible to enhance a body's protein quality control mechanisms to maintain proteostasis and potentially mitigate age-related protein aggregation and related diseases, thus supporting overall bodily health.

- **ALTERED CELLULAR COMMUNICATION** — It should go without saying that humans are multicellular organisms. It's estimated that our bodies are composed of about 37.2 trillion cells. But for our bodies to function as systems, these cells must communicate with each other. To do so, our cells send out tiny chemical signals that act on the receptors on other cells. Scientists classify these signals according to the distance between the signaling cell and the target cell so that autocrine signals are produced by a cell and received by its own receptors, paracrine signals are produced by a cell to target nearby cells, and endocrine signals target cells that are farther away. NAD plays a pivotal role in regulating these signals, so when NAD declines, communication can become fuzzy. Signals are not sent at the proper time or fail to reach their target. At times, a targeted cell simply doesn't respond. Without functional intercellular communication, systems break down and disease sets in. Perhaps the prototypical "failed signal" disease is diabetes. Normally, the pancreas releases insulin to signal the liver, muscle, and fat cells to store sugar for later use. In type I diabetes, cells in the pancreas do not produce the insulin signal. In type II diabetes, the signal is reduced and cannot be received. In either case, sugar accumulates to toxic levels in the blood. By optimizing NAD levels, it is possible to help restore proper cellular communication and signaling pathways, potentially mitigating age-related cellular dysfunction, and promoting healthier aging.

Now that we understand a little about how NAD+ operates on the cellular level, we can look closely at how it supports organs and systems, and how that support manifests in improved health.

CHAPTER 8

THE PROMISE OF NAD

"Embracing this path, we are like newborn children. We are in natural harmony with all creatures, bringing harm to none. Our body is soft and flexible, yet strong."

—Lao-Tzu, *Tao Te Ching*

In the following section, I explore a number of stubborn maladies that impede our health, accelerate aging, and invite disease. I call them stubborn, because science has not definitively solved the puzzle of why these conditions arise or how to overcome them. We know a little, and that knowledge has helped some people who suffer from these conditions to improve and regain their health. But for the vast majority of sufferers, these conditions linger and worsen, until they become the defining characteristic of their lives.

But the good news is that NAD research, which has only just begun, provides solid grounds for optimism. NAD depletion may be a key factor in the emergence of various maladies, and so, NAD optimization might be a way to "turn back the clock," or as we say in the digital age, "reboot and refresh." In this section, I do not want to overpromise. But I will cite reliable scientific studies, along with individual testimonials, which strongly suggest that people suffering from these stubborn conditions can get noticeable, even profound, relief by optimizing their NAD levels.

Because you, dear reader, might only be interested in exploring the sections that pertain to your symptoms, or those of a loved one, I present this breakdown of this chapter's contents.

- **Brain health**
    - Brain fog
    - Addiction
    - Symptoms of trauma
    - Neurodegenerative diseases (e.g., Alzheimer's, Parkinson's)
    - Autism
- **Oxidative stress: the dysfunction behind far-too-many metabolic disorders**
    - Cardiovascular disease
    - Inflammatory pain
    - Insulin resistance
    - Arthritis
- **Sexual health, increased libido, and extended fertility**
    - Libido
    - Female reproduction

- **Sleep disorders and chronic fatigue**
  - Insomnia
  - Chronic Fatigue Syndrome
- **Cancer**
- **Healthy vision**
  - Age-related macular degeneration
- **Allergies and asthma**
- **Strength and stamina**
  - Musculature

Now, with further ado, let's perform a deeper dive into stubborn maladies and the promise of NAD.

Brain Health

Let's start with a subject that's on everyone's mind.

In January 2023, the Dana Foundation[15] published the results of a survey on brain health. The Foundation polled more than 2,200 Americans and found that 82 percent claimed that they or someone close to them had experienced at least one brain health condition. The leading conditions cited were:

- **DEPRESSION** — 55 percent of respondents
- **ALZHEIMER'S DISEASE OR DEMENTIA** — 48 percent

15 *https://dana.org/article/survey-finds-brain-health-is-a-top-priority-for-americans/*

- **SUBSTANCE USE DISORDER OR ADDICTION** — 42 percent
- **GENERALIZED ANXIETY DISORDER** — 42 percent

Moreover, The National Institute of Mental Health reports that nearly one in five adults and nearly one in two adolescents live with a mental illness, such as anxiety or depression. The National Institute of Neurological Disorders and Stroke also reports that one in five adults lives with a neurological illness, such as dementia or multiple sclerosis. The reasons for poor brain health are both somatic and psychological. Causes vary, including physical trauma, emotional trauma, infectious disease, degenerative disease, and organic pathologies that science cannot explain.

The brain is the "seat of consciousness," defining who we are as individuals. Yet, despite being the most important organ in the human body, it is the least understood. Sadly, when the brain is not healthy, life can devolve into a nightmare. Therefore, whether we are talking about mental and psychological health or the somatic health of the brain as an organ, we must address our current crisis in brain health. And NAD+ optimization might be an important part of the solution.

Recently, the noted brain health expert, Dr. James Goodwin, the author of *Supercharge Your Brain*, was suffering from debilitating fatigue. He took *Jinfiniti*'s NAD test, which revealed that his NAD+ levels were severely deficient. As he explains:

> *"Over the last year, I started experiencing really debilitating fatigue in the afternoon. About six months ago, I did the NAD test and got shockingly low results coming in deficient. I'm perfectly healthy. I don't have any diagnosed medical conditions. I exercise*

regularly, I eat well, and I'm not overweight. I was so appalled and determined to start taking the supplements regularly.

"Two weeks into taking the NAD supplement, the fatigue disappeared. I was absolutely astonished. I'm not going to stop taking the supplements to see if the fatigue comes back. I'd recommend the Vitality boost to anyone who needs extra energy."

If the Director of the Brain Health Network in London now believes in NAD+ optimization, who am I to contradict him?

We know that NAD is essential to almost every cellular process in the human body, and what cellular processes are more urgent than those that happen within our cranium? Could underperformance, sluggishness, injury, illness, and impairment be alleviated with NAD+? A recent article published in *Science Direct* reviewed 20 "peer-reviewed, published preclinical studies evaluating NR on various parameters of brain health and neurodegeneration." NR, as we've noted, is an effective NAD+ precursor. This study concluded that NR is a demonstrably safe compound, and that "oral NR supplementation has been shown to be successful in multiple preclinical models of neurodegeneration and brain function, [thus] there is ample evidence to support clinical evaluation of NR as a support for brain health."

Given the research, I believe NAD optimization can be a useful tool to remediate a variety of conditions, including:

"BRAIN FOG" — This mental fuzziness is characterized by confusion, forgetfulness, and a lack of focus. Causes include overwork, lack of sleep, stress, a sedentary lifestyle, and too much time spent on a computer. It is also related to unhealthy conditions, such as obesity and diabetes. On a cellular level, brain fog has been linked to inflammation and hormonal imbalances, conditions which NAD+ directly impacts. As we have noted, NAD plays a key role in cellular health by guarding against mitochondrial dysfunction and oxidative stress. In brain cells particularly, NAD boosts the production of PGC-1-alpha, a protein that protects brain cells. Additionally, NAD acts as a neurotransmitter. As we've discussed, this requires electric charges, and NAD+ often supplies the spark. Think about how many times you've seen an illustration of someone getting a bright idea, and the artist has placed a light bulb over their head. Our brains need the positive charge of NAD+. To put this in perspective, your brain is only three percent of your body weight, but it uses 20 percent of your energy in calories. Therefore, when your body is deficient in NAD, your brain is especially depleted. Don't let low NAD be a drain on your brain!

Moreover, if your NAD is so low that you're foggy headed, what do you imagine is happening in your other tissues? Chances are, you've got additional symptoms often linked to brain fog, such as:

- Impaired sleep or insomnia
- Headaches
- Fatigue
- Poor memory
- Mood swings
- Irritability
- Low motivation
- Excessive absences from work or social commitments
- Mildly depression or chronic sadness

- Hypothyroidism
- Sjögren's syndrome, a chronic inflammatory autoimmune disease

Anecdotally, we have seen many clients achieve significant reductions in brain fog and fatigue when they boost their NAD levels with our state-of-the-art, high-performing supplements.

ADDICTION — Cravings and dependencies live in the brain. Addictions take hold because the addictive substances interfere with the way neurons send, receive, and process signals via neurotransmitters. The chemical structure of certain drugs mimics that of a natural neurotransmitter in the body. Thus, drugs attach to and activate neurons. This mimicry creates an abnormal norm, altering the way messages are sent through the neural network. As we've discussed, NAD+ is vital for regulating cell signaling. It's logical, therefore, to suppose that NAD+ could restore normal functioning to neural pathways that have been disrupted.

In early studies and data tracking, the Springfield Wellness Center (the first NAD+ clinic in America) found that NAD+ therapy has a nearly 400 percent better success rate than conventional drug rehab practices, because NAD+ infusions help the brain chemistry rebalance while reducing or eliminating cravings for addictive substances.

NAD+ IV coupled with NAC and other vital nutrients and minerals were observed to help rewire neural pathways, detox patients, optimize mitochondrial energy, and eliminate chemical cravings. Two years after treatment, participants in the study, who began with very high cravings for drugs or alcohol, still had essentially no cravings. That elimination of cravings is the Holy Grail of recovery.

SYMPTOMS OF TRAUMA — Different types of trauma can impact brain function. First, there is physical trauma, as we see in traumatic brain injury, where blunt force, concussive force, penetration of the cranium, or excessive shaking has actually destroyed tissue. Second, there is the trauma of emotional overload from circumstances that are highly stressful or terrifying. In either case, it is not just the mind that is affected; the traumatic event dramatically alters the structure of the brain. The result is post-traumatic stress disorder (PTSD)—a syndrome consisting of various cognitive, physical, and psychological symptoms—depression, or chronic anxiety. We cannot go back in time and prevent the injury event, so how do we heal our brains and return to sound mental, psychological, and somatic health?

A couple of incidents that clients have brought to our attention strongly suggest that NAD+ supplementation can be an effective therapy for the physical and psychological symptoms we typically ascribe to PTSD. This first account comes from an email of November 20, 2023, from a reputable professional, who is also a distributor of our NAD+ supplements:

> *I want to share a very important issue with you. A woman reached us 2-3 weeks ago and shared the situation of her child. 1.5 years ago, while her son was playing at school, he fell into a well, and when he was taken out of the well and brought to the hospital, he was dead. He was later revived with heart massage and remained in intensive care for 6 months. During this process, he can only move his eyes. He can neither speak nor move.*

Later, the doctors tell the woman that there is nothing to be done and that they should take the child home. As a last resort, They go to Dr. Ender Saraç, you know, we introduced him to our NAD test. He applies our NAD test to the child and gives supplements. They use it regularly, then the mother contacted us and said that this supplement is vital for her child, and she should definitely take it. When we asked him why it was important, she said that thanks to NAD, her son was now walking and no one, including the doctors, could believe it. So, the child who only moved his eyes is now walking. I wanted to share this with you. We think it's a miracle. We would appreciate, if you could please give us your thoughts on what we should do about this issue, because we need to process this incident.

Best regards,
Hakan ŞAHİNOĞLU
Uluslararası İlişkiler Müdürü
International Business Manager

This child obviously sustained intense physical and emotional trauma. The symptoms described indicate the kind of emotional overload that induces shock leading to neurological impairment. Loss of motor skills is common in patients with traumatic brain injury and/or PTSD, and these patients face a long, torturous road to recovery, which is generally incomplete. The rapid progress this child made is truly remarkable, which suggests that deeper inquiry into the effectiveness of NAD+ supplementation as treatment is warranted.

Shocks like the one this child experienced can also lead to profound depression, which, according to conventional medical understanding, has no cure. Some patients improve with antidepressant medications but can't discontinue those meds without a recurrence of symptoms. And, all the while, they must deal with side effects, including the often-tragic suicidal ideation. However, in my opinion, informed by thousands of clinical studies, many diseases and ailments conventional medicine calls lost causes actually have potential solutions. In our labs, we have seen many, many clients experience significant improvements in their mental health after optimizing their NAD levels.

I'll let our client, Sarah, tell her story:

> *"For over two years, my mental health suffered. I felt like my brain was broken. I battled high levels of anxiety, having panic attacks three times a week, I felt fatigued all the time and needed 400 mg of caffeine and two naps per day just to function. It felt like a single setback could slide me off the cliff.*
>
> *"Initially, I did a big round of NAD IV, which was $4000, but I was desperate. It gave me a lot of energy and mental lift, but it wasn't sustainable. A few months later, I was feeling the same. And then I discovered* Jinfiniti*. My NAD levels were sorely deficient.*
>
> *"Within several months of taking Vitality boost, my energy is much higher, my mental health and anxiety is so much better, and I've even lost some of the unwanted stubborn weight that wouldn't go away. And my NAD levels are now optimal at 55.4 thanks to* Vitality Boost.
>
> *"My husband and I feel we have our lives back and I know* Jinfiniti*'s been a huge part of that."*

As a trained scientist, I know better than to draw sweeping conclusions from anecdotes, no matter how compelling the individual facts might be. But from what I know about cell functions, I believe there is great potential for NAD+ to assist in recovery from PTSD, depression, and chronic anxiety. I look forward to future clinical trials with cohorts of patients suffering from these conditions.

ALZHEIMER'S, PARKINSON'S, AND OTHER NEURODEGENERATIVE DISEASES — Every older adult occasionally has a "senior moment." But when age combines with metabolic deficiencies, that's a recipe for severe, disabling pathology. For decades, Alzheimer's disease has been seen as a slow-motion death sentence, where patients lose a bit of themselves every day. Parkinson's disease captures the body, transforming it into a torture chamber for patients who lose control of their impulses and are subjected to constant tremors. However, early research indicates that NAD can effectively treat some of the most prominent neurodegenerative diseases. Brain chemistry, cellular signaling, and cell function—specifically metabolic processes—are central issues with neurological diseases, and NAD plays a key role.

In August 2022[16], the Swiss journal MDPI published a review of scientific literature by Jared M. Campbell of the Graduate School of Biomedical Engineering, at the University of New South Wales in Sydney, Australia. Entitled, *Supplementation with NAD+ and Its Precursors to Prevent Cognitive Decline across Disease Contexts*, the study examined findings related to a broad range of neurodegenerative diseases. Campbell concludes that "A large body of preclinical research supports the potential effectiveness of NAD+ precursor supplementation

16 *Campbell, J.M. Supplementation with NAD+ and Its Precursors to Prevent Cognitive Decline across Disease Contexts. Nutrients 2022, 14, 3231. https:// doi.org/10.3390/nu14153231*

for preserving cognitive health across a variety of disease contexts, with the strongest evidence presented for Alzheimer's disease and other forms of dementia."

Additionally, experts at the Springfield Wellness Center have treated many patients with dementia or Parkinson's. When these patients receive NAD+ treatments, their symptoms often go into remission. Of course, the earlier the treatment begins, the better and quicker the results. Unfortunately, researchers have not conducted enough clinical trials to test NAD's effects on neurodegenerative diseases for anyone to make empirical claims in favor of NAD, but we are excited for what future studies might show.

In the meantime, there is nothing stopping any concerned individual from trying NAD optimization for brain health. However, we suggest you also supplement nutrients with proven efficacy, including:

- **VITAMIN D** — This essential nutrient, celebrated for building strong bones and warding off seasonal affective disorder during the winter months, also plays a vital role in maintaining healthy cognitive function. Vitamin D deficiencies may accelerate aging and make the body vulnerable to a range of debilitating conditions, including infection, osteoporosis, heart disease, type II diabetes, and cancer.
- **CREATINE** — This natural compound, made from three animo acids, is found in meat and fish, and also made by the human body in the liver, kidneys, and pancreas. Creatine gets converted into creatine phosphate or phosphocreatine and stored in the muscles, where it is used for energy. Creatine's most important function is to

serve as a battery or reserve for the energy-storage molecule ATP. Additionally, creatine increases muscle mass and improves brain function.

- **EPA FATTY ACIDS** — Anyone who might have told you that "Fish is brain food," might have been referencing eicosapentaenoic acid (EPA), one of several omega-3 fatty acids found in cold-water fatty fish, such as salmon. Known as "healthy brain fats," these substances support mental health and longevity. Dr. Andrew Huberman, the noted Stanford neuroscientist speaks candidly about how 1000 mg of EPA fatty acids have the equivalent effect of an anti-depressant for more than 70 percent of people!

Any program to heal the brain and increase mental health should also attempt to minimize unhealthy foods that literally act as neurotoxins. These include conventionally fried foods, refined sugar, alcohol, and processed foods.

AUTISM — Autism spectrum disorder (ASD) is a complex condition characterized by problems with social interaction, verbal, and nonverbal communication, and repetitive or restrictive behavior. Autism is regarded as a spectrum, because the symptoms vary widely in type and intensity from one individual to another. Researchers have not determined exactly what causes autism, though genetic and environmental factors are thought to play a role. Autism is a lifelong condition, presenting multiple, ongoing challenges to autistic individuals and their families. Certain therapies have been shown to alleviate some of the difficulties for some individuals, but nothing approaching a cure has been suggested.

Might NAD+ supplementation help in cases of autism? Recent research shows some promise, but before we get into those studies, let us examine more closely the possible causes of autism spectrum disorder.

According to the National Institutes of Health[17], genetic mutations are present in most people with autism. However, these mutations occur in different genes and in different combinations. Thus, "Not everyone with autism has changes in every gene that scientists have linked to ASD." To further complicate matters, "Many people without autism ... also have ... genetic mutations that scientists have linked to autism." The variety of genetic mutations may account for the broad spectrum of the disorder. Scientists also believe that individuals who are genetically susceptible to ADS may develop the disorder due to environmental factors, such as infection or exposure to a toxin. NIH firmly denies that vaccines are an environmental factor that triggers ASD.

Additional biological factors that may lead to autism might include:

- Problems with brain connections or the growth in certain areas of the brain
- Metabolic problems
- Immune system problems

17 *https://www.nichd.nih.gov/health/topics/autism/conditioninfo/causes*

The organization *Autism Speaks*[18] cites the following risk factors for developing ASD:

- Advanced age of either parent
- Pregnancy and birth complications, such as extreme prematurity, low birth weight, multiple pregnancies
- Pregnancies spaced less than one year apart

Another putative authority, Total Regenerative Medical Health[19], an organization that treats autistic individuals with NAD infusion, adds "Maternal obesity, diabetes, or immune system disorders" to the list of factors.

We have already seen that many of these factors—genetic mutation, metabolic illnesses, immune system problems, and parental fertility—relate to NAD+ under other circumstances. NAD+ helps cell replication to ensure that DNA is not damaged, and mutations do not take place. When metabolic diseases are present, NAD+ is generally depleted. The same can be said for immune system failure. And we know that NAD+ helps improve fertility in older female mice, which suggests it could be efficacious for mature women. Citing "maternal obesity, diabetes, or immune system disorders" as risk factors is very interesting, because this suggests the mother's NAD+ levels are almost certainly not what they should be, which suggests the child's womb environment might not provide sufficient levels of NAD+ for healthy growth.

18 *https://www.autismspeaks.org/what-causes-autism*

19 *https://totalrmh.com/what-we-treat/autism/*

Based on these risk factors, my instinct tells me that prospective parents should consider NAD+ supplementation ahead of (and during) pregnancy as a preventative measure. Could NAD+ help prevent genetic mutations that invite autism? The question is certainly worth asking. Especially when authorities, such as *Autism Speaks*, tell us that "Prenatal vitamins containing folic acid, before and at conception and through pregnancy" decrease the risk of autism. Folic acid, also known as Vitamin B9, is part of the B complex, which includes Niacin or B3. As the Linus Pauling Institute states, "Niacin or vitamin B3 is a water-soluble vitamin used by the body to form the nicotinamide coenzyme, NAD+."

All the B vitamins perform specific functions, but also work together on virtually all metabolic and developmental processes within the body: energy production, cell division, cell replication, growth, etc. Thus, taking a B vitamin complex would help cells produce more NAD+. But if that is the goal, why not just supplement the precursors of NAD?

Along these lines, we might also wonder if some type of supplementation might alleviate some autism symptoms. In fact, research into the role of mitochondrial damage in autism patients suggests that such a program might be beneficial. According to an article on fxMedicine.com[20], there is "evidence [which] suggests there is a subset of ASD individuals with concomitant mitochondrial dysfunction (MD)." As we've already discussed, impairment of mitochondrial activity negatively impacts energy metabolism, forming free radicals which produce oxidative stress. The article doesn't mention NAD+

20 *https://www.fxmedicine.com.au/blog-post/mitochondrial-dysfunction-autism-spectrum-disorders*

by name but notes that "When there are optimal levels of endogenous antioxidant substances and enzymes in the mitochondrial membrane, including glutathione, vitamins C and E and superoxide dismutase (SOD), the detrimental impact of ROS is restricted." In other words, these particular autism patients were under oxidative stress, and thus, needed a nutritional intervention to overcome the problems posed by the mitochondrial damage. (And we have seen that in other situations, NAD+ relieves oxidative stress.)

This study concludes that ASD-MD individuals gained some benefit from supplementing "essential fatty acids, coenzyme Q10, carnitine, carnosine, and vitamins B1, B2, B3, B12 (methylcobalamin), C and folic or folinic acid." Those benefits included "improvements in muscle tone, intellectual disability, cognition, childhood autism rating scale, clinical global impressions scores, ETC complex I activity, glutathione concentrations and reduced levels of Clostridia-derived metabolites." These improvements were achieved without supplementing one of the most essential compounds for mitochondrial function: NAD+. It seems natural to ask, "Would the results have been even better, if they'd optimized for NAD?"

Animal tests also suggest that NAD+ can be efficacious for ASD. A study published in *Scientific Reports*[21] for June 2020 was entitled, *Nicotinamide riboside supplementation corrects deficits in oxytocin, sociability, and anxiety of CD157 mutants in a mouse model of autism spectrum disorder*. The researchers studied mice

21 *Gerasimenko, M., Cherepanov, S.M., Furuhara, K. et al. Nicotinamide riboside supplementation corrects deficits in oxytocin, sociability and anxiety of CD157 mutants in a mouse model of autism spectrum disorder. Sci Rep 10, 10035 (2020). https://doi.org/10.1038/s41598-019-57236-7*

that were missing a gene, which effectively gave them ASD. The researchers observed that NR, an efficacious NAD+ precursor, "corrects social deficits and fearful and anxiety-like behaviors in [ADS] males." The results of this study suggest that "elevating NAD levels with nicotinamide riboside may allow [autistic] animals … to overcome these deficits and function more normally."

This is by no means sufficient evidence to conclude that NAD+ can alleviate autism in humans. However, given the absence of effective remedies and the safety profile for this natural compound, parents searching for answers have turned to NAD+ optimization for whatever benefits their children might derive. One example is three-year-old Corbin, who has engaged in a wide range of therapies that include detoxes, 40x hyperbaric oxygen therapy sessions using a 2ATA hyperbaric chamber, chelation therapy, reverse osmosis water filtration, ABA therapy, speech therapy, and occupational therapy.

Corbin's mother heard me speak at an Autism Health Summit and decided to try our product, *Vitality Boost*. In an email to me a short time later, March 2024, his mother explained that she and her husband, as well as the boy's therapists and teacher noted the following changes:

- **INCREASED FOCUS AND ENGAGEMENT** — Corbin has been able to sit attentively during therapy sessions and activities, as well as with his teacher during mealtimes.
- **IMPROVED FINE MOTOR SKILLS** — He has demonstrated the ability to put individual popsicle sticks inside a toothbrush holder, indicating progress in his fine motor abilities.

- **ENHANCED COMMUNICATION SKILLS** — Despite being mostly non-verbal, Corbin has shown progress in communication by interrupting his teacher to get her attention and indicating his wants and needs more clearly.
- **INCREASED INDEPENDENCE** — Corbin has started opening his snack containers and lunch box, showing improved independence in daily tasks.
- **IMPROVED RESPONSIVENESS** — He now responds with "yeah" when asked if he wants something, indicating better understanding and communication.
- **BETTER UNDERSTANDING OF VERBAL COMMANDS** — Corbin can now follow verbal commands like putting his shoes on, demonstrating improved listening skills.
- **INCREASED AFFECTION AND SOCIAL ENGAGEMENT** — He has been more affectionate and cuddly, initiating play more often with his parents and seeking approval through eye contact.
- **EXPANDED VOCABULARY** — Corbin has started saying new words and phrases like "Peek-a-boo," "I wake up," and "I pee-pee," showing progress in his language development.
- **IMPROVED BEHAVIOR IN PUBLIC SETTINGS** — He displayed patience and waiting behavior at the splash pad, a notable improvement from previous behaviors of attempting to run away.

More research is needed, but we are so excited about the potential of NAD+ alleviating symptoms of autism that we are launching our own study, which we've dubbed the Autism Warrior Project. As I've mentioned several times, I am a data-driven scientist, so I want to study this problem in full detail. However, for now, if you are the parent of an autistic child, I can highly recommend *Vitality Boost* to support your child's overall health and well-being.

Oxidative Stress: the Dysfunction Behind Far-Too-Many Metabolic Disorders

Suppose there was one simple supplement that could guard against neurodegenerative diseases (Parkinson's disease, Alzheimer's disease, ALS, multiple sclerosis, and dementia), high cholesterol, heart failure, heart attack, hypertension, stroke, atherosclerosis, diabetes, chronic pain due to inflammation, and other obesity-related disorders. Would you take it? All of the above conditions are consequences of oxidative stress. We've touched on this condition briefly already, but its prevalence in our society and its dire consequences merit a fuller explanation.

Cellular health relies on a balance between compounds that incite activity and those that suppress it. When that balance is off, our cell processes can become overactive, creating stress that damages cells and causes cascading health problems. This is what happens with the condition we call oxidative stress.

Oxidation is a beneficial process. Simply put, it is the cell's process of respiration. Most of us understand human respiration in highly simplistic terms: we inhale oxygen and exhale carbon dioxide. This happens because the air we breathe in undergoes a chemical change within our cells. We "use up" the oxygen and expel its byproducts.

On the cellular level, oxidation involves the transfer of electrons, as nutrients are turned into energy. Within individual cells, oxygen combines with glucose to produce energy in the form of adenosine triphosphate (ATP), and the cell expels carbon dioxide and water. Thus, glucose is oxidized, and oxygen is reduced. To keep this process in a healthy balance, cells contain both free radicals, which encourage oxidation, and antioxidant defense mechanisms, which keep the process in check.

Oxidative stress occurs when the free radicals overwhelm the antioxidant defenses. Free radicals are molecules that contain atoms with unpaired (i.e., extra) electrons. Too many free radicals mean too many extra electrons driving oxidation up to unhealthy levels. The body uses antioxidants to suppress the free radicals, but these can be in short supply, especially if an individual maintains a poor diet, is exposed to toxic chemicals, smokes, or consumes too much alcohol.

Common antioxidants which combat free radicals include Vitamins C and E, glutathione, beta-carotene, and plant estrogens called phytoestrogens. Supplementing these compounds can fight oxidative stress. However, another complicating factor is that our bodies lose their ability to fight free radicals with age.

This age-related inability seems to involve the mitochondria, those tiny organelles which are the engines of cell activity. Free radicals can interfere with the mitochondrial processes, so more free radicals are produced, and new cells are more likely to have damaged DNA. The result is accelerated aging and greater susceptibility to age-related illnesses, including those we mentioned which are related to oxidative stress. Optimizing levels of NAD+ can restore a variety of mitochondrial functions, thereby reducing oxidative stress and its consequences.

Let's discuss a few of the most serious consequences of unaddressed oxidative stress.

CARDIOVASCULAR DISEASE — Heart disease[22] is the number one killer of Americans, so any factor that contributes to this condition deserves intensive scrutiny. For quite a while, medical science has recognized a relationship between oxidative stress and cardiac pathologies. Starting in the 1990s, researchers observed a correlation between high inflammation levels and an increased risk of heart attacks and strokes. (Inflammation, which we explore in greater detail below, is a consequence of oxidative stress.) However, doctors continued to believe that the major culprit in heart disease was artery-clogging cholesterol. To combat this villain, pharmaceutical companies developed statin drugs, designed to reduce LDL, the bad type of cholesterol. Then, in 2008, the JUPITER study found that statin drugs also reduced the rate of heart attack and stroke in older adults with normal LDL cholesterol but elevated inflammatory markers. As it turns out, statin drugs also have anti-inflammatory effects. So, why were statin drugs beneficial? Were they reducing LDL or inflammation? That was unclear.

But in 2017, the CANTOS trial demonstrated that targeting inflammation, independent of cholesterol, reduced the likelihood of future heart attack or stroke by 15 percent in subjects with a history of those conditions. Also, by targeting inflammation, the need for major surgical interventions decreased by 30 percent. It became apparent that inflammation was a significant factor in heart disease, which should not be surprising,

22 *https://www.rupahealth.com/post/inflammation-and-heart-disease-a-functional-medicine-approach-to-prevention-and-treatment*

given the destructive consequences of even low-grade chronic inflammation for affected tissues.

Controlling inflammation with pharmaceuticals was a step forward. But why not go a step further and prevent that inflammation by eliminating oxidative stress? We have every reason to believe that optimized NAD+ can help in this regard.

INFLAMMATORY PAIN — As we get older, we are more likely to experience pain without an apparent cause. You did no heavy lifting, yet you have a flare-up of sciatica. Yesterday, you did nothing more than soft toss a Nerf football to your grandson, but today you can't pick up your arm. These types of pains, due to inflammation, have their root cause in oxidative stress.

Under oxidative stress, your body knows that cells are damaged, and it initiates an immune response. This is all very healthy. However, since oxidative stress is a chronic condition, that immune response persists and goes into overdrive, producing debilitating pain. Now you've got chronic low-grade inflammation, which can lead to arthritis, diabetes, cancer, cardiovascular disease and more. It can also contribute to neurodegenerative diseases like Alzheimer's and Parkinson's.

You can treat the symptoms with ice packs, heating pads, Ibuprofen, and rest. But what you really need is to attack the root cause through lifestyle modification and targeted supplements.

ARTHRITIS — As we just mentioned, chronic inflammation can lead to arthritis, which is characterized by painful swelling in the joints, along with stiffness and a loss in the range of motion. There are two main forms of arthritis that attack joints in different ways. Osteoarthritis (OA) is the most prevalent joint degenerative disease. It causes irreversible structural and functional changes to the joints. OA is a major cause of disability and reduced life expectancy in older adults. Rheumatoid arthritis (RA) is an immune system response that attacks the lining of the joint capsule, a durable membrane that encloses all the joint parts. When this synovial membrane remains inflamed, cartilage and bone within the joint are destroyed. To make matters worse, arthritis sufferers are also likely to develop other debilitating conditions, such as cardiovascular disease, lung disease, and lymphoma.

Despite the prevalence of arthritis in the United States, there are no medications that can effectively reverse the disease. What arthritis sufferers must do is reverse oxidative stress. This requires lifestyle modification along with supplements that can eliminate free radicals and reduce inflammation. But on the cellular level, we know we must improve cell functions, and that starts with optimizing our NAD+!

INSULIN RESISTANCE — Insulin is a hormone produced by the pancreas, which aids in our metabolism. When we digest food, our body converts nutrients into dietary sugars, which enter the blood stream. The pancreas responds by releasing insulin to signal our cells to open up and absorb the blood glucose and convert it to energy. Insulin resistance, also known as prediabetes, is a condition where the cells do not respond adequately to the signal. Blood glucose remains at high levels, and the pancreas continues to pump out insulin until the organ exhausts itself. When the pancreas no longer produces insulin, diabetes sets in.

Although anyone can become insulin resistant, certain health factors increase the likelihood of the condition arising, including excess weight, a family history of type II diabetes, smoking, and being age 45 or older. Certain medications, such as steroids, anti-psychotics, and HIV drugs, can cause insulin resistance. The condition is also prevalent in individuals who suffer from medical conditions, such as obstructive sleep apnea, fatty liver disease, polycystic ovarian syndrome, Cushing's syndrome (overproduction of the stress hormone cortisol), and lipodystrophy syndromes (conditions that cause fat loss in some areas accompanied by gains somewhere else).

Many people with insulin resistance do not manifest overt symptoms. But common signs include weight gain around the waist, such that a man's waistline exceeds 40 inches or a woman's 35 inches, skin tags, *acanthosis nigricans* (dark, velvety patches in areas where the skin is folded or creased), blood pressure reading of 130 over 80 or higher, a high blood glucose level, high "bad" cholesterol, and low "good" cholesterol.

As an unhealthy metabolic syndrome, insulin resistance can lead to serious disease if untreated. Complications can include severe blood sugar abnormalities, type II diabetes, heart attack, stroke, kidney disease, vision problems, cancer, and Alzheimer's disease. Conventional treatments include dietary and lifestyle modifications. A healthy diet of lean protein, fresh fruits and vegetables, nuts, and whole grains, along with portion control, can bring weight down and help balance the metabolism. Regular exercise, at least a half hour a day, five days a week, can help to restore balance. Unfortunately, insulin resistance is a stubborn condition. It dampens our mood and lowers our energy, so it becomes difficult to maintain a healthy regimen. If you are constantly tired, and your new diet and exercise program don't seem to be helping you shed pounds or regain your energy, it's easy to slip back into established patterns. Pretty soon, you're back on the couch with a bucket of KFC. This is why too many individuals wind up relying on prescription medications, which alleviate symptoms but do not address the root causes. Thus, a patient can delay complications but cannot hide from them for long. As Dr. Lustig has said, "You can't outrun a bad diet," especially from your couch.

Fortunately, early studies of the effects of NAD+ optimization on insulin resistance are encouraging. In November 2020, the *Journal of Diabetes Investigation*[23] published the results of a "randomized, placebo-controlled, double-blind trial," which examined the effects of NMN supplementation on muscle insulin sensitivity in "postmenopausal women with prediabetes who are overweight or obese." The researchers found "clinically relevant" improvement in muscle insulin sensitivity, which was "similar to the improvement observed after ~10 percent weight loss and after 12 weeks of treatment with the insulin sensitizing agent troglitazone in people with obesity." In other words, NAD+ optimization got similar results without requiring weight loss or three months of prescription medication.

More recently, researchers from the University of Washington[24] found that supplementing healthy, middle-aged adults with a formulation of NAD+ precursors "significantly increases blood levels of NAD+" and "lowers blood glucose while leaving insulin levels unaltered." The researchers also noted improvements in stress hormone levels.

---

23 *https://www.ncbi.nlm.nih.gov/pmc/articles/PMC8550608/*

24 *https://www.nmn.com/news/nad-booster-riagev-improves-insulin-sensitivity-and-stress-hormone-levels*

Finally, in March 2022[25], the journal *Nutrition and Metabolism* published a meta-analysis of the *Effects of NAD+ precursor supplementation on glucose and lipid metabolism in humans*. The article concludes that "the supplement of NAD+precursors seems to have little effect on healthy people, but it has a significant beneficial effect on patients with cardiovascular disease and dyslipidemia." By dyslipidemia, doctors mean a condition of abnormally elevated cholesterol or fats in the blood. Dyslipidemia raises the risks of blocked arteries, heart attacks, stroke, or other circulatory problems, especially in smokers. Dyslipidemia in adults is yet another consequence of obesity, an unhealthy diet, and a sedentary lifestyle.

As mentioned earlier, insulin resistance can be difficult to defeat, because it's hard to get low-energy people to make the lifestyle choices that lead to better health. It's a proverbial "journey of a thousand miles" demanded of someone who would rather take a nap. There's a similar hurdle for people suffering from heart ailments, inflammatory pain, and arthritis. Doctors can tell their patients that "motion is the potion," but when every movement is torture, they're going to remain very still. Fortunately, NAD+ optimization makes very little demand on these individuals. Take a supplement twice a day, and let your energy improve. Now it's much easier to contemplate a change of diet and a few minutes on the treadmill. All of a sudden, people who were intractable in their bad habits are making incremental lifestyle improvements, moving with greater ease, shedding pounds, and maintaining a positive

25 *Zhong, O., Wang, J., Tan, Y. et al. Effects of NAD+ precursor supplementation on glucose and lipid metabolism in humans: a meta-analysis. Nutr Metab (Lond) 19, 20 (2022). https://doi.org/10.1186/s12986-022-00653-9*

outlook. To borrow from Lao Tzu, the journey of a thousand miles begins with NAD!

Sexual Health, Increased Libido, and Extended Fertility

One of the happier discoveries our clients are making about NAD+ is that it rejuvenates their sex life. There are a host of reasons why this is the case:

- **GREATER ENERGY** — Romance within a marriage can fizzle when spouses are working long hours then slumping at the end of a busy day. Physical fatigue often quashes any desire for intimacy.
- **BETTER MOOD** — When you have more energy, your mood is brighter. You're more playful and affectionate with your partner, which can lead to satisfying results.
- **MORE CONFIDENCE** — Even if you are married, initiating a romantic encounter requires confidence. This is especially true for men, whose reticence can make create difficulties with performance. Since "Faint heart never won fair lady," the confidence one gains from NAD+ optimization can make a great difference.
- **HORMONAL HEIGHTS** — Libido is linked to hormones, which are in short supply when you're chronically exhausted, but flourish when your NAD+ is optimized.
- **BETTER ABLE TO CONNECT** — Intimacy is about connection. When you're feeling depleted, you collapse into yourself and your ability to connect with others weakens. If you're foggy headed, you're not fully present to your partner. The greater mental clarity you derive from NAD+ primes you for intimacy.

I continually hear from *Jinfiniti* clients who report increased libido and greater sexual satisfaction after using *Vitality Boost*. One such client is Alina, a native of Romania and a dentist, who is now 50 years old. When she was 48, she had her NAD+ level tested, recording a 19, which is basically what we would expect from an 80-year-old. At the time, Alina was probably 50 pounds overweight and complained of being terribly fatigued all the time. Her NAD+ level quickly reached 50, then after a couple of months soared to 70. Alina actually tapered back the dosage because she felt had too much energy.

At that point, Alina started giving *Vitality Boost* to her husband, who was 18 years her senior. He is a semi-retired lawyer, who is healthy and active for his age. But since taking *Vitality Boost*, he has much more energy and stamina. Recently, Alina mentioned that "the blood is going," and her husband is "horny like crazy." Not that Alina minds. She says that in her culture, physical intimacy in a marriage is highly valued, so couples should not curtail lovemaking, even as they mature. She's happy to share that she and her husband are having sex three times a day!

An active sex life can do wonders for a marriage, but let's not forget nature's purpose for making sex so pleasurable. This is the means by which humanity propagates and survives as a species. So, we have to wonder if NAD+ has a part to play in reproduction as well.

FEMALE FERTILITY — Not long ago, various sources were issuing dire warnings of global overpopulation leading to a depletion of resources and mass starvation. In 1968, Dr. Paul

Ehrlich[26], an entomologist at Stanford University, released a book entitled *The Population Bomb*, whose first sentence sent shockwaves down his readers' spines: "The battle to feed all of humanity is over." According to Ehrlich, we had already lost that battle, and in subsequent decades hundreds of millions of people would die of starvation. Ehrlich promoted his book at every opportunity, including a segment of *The Tonight Show* with Johnny Carson. In a subsequent interview, he told *CBS News*, "Sometime in the next 15 years, the end will come. And by 'the end' I mean an utter breakdown of the capacity of the planet to support humanity."

Hollywood, eager as ever to capitalize on an apocalyptic nightmare, produced dystopian films, such as *Soylent Green*, where the exploding human population had ravaged all resources, so that even the seas were barren. With animals and plant life extinct, humanity was reduced to eating each other.

Fast-forward 55 years, and not only was *The Population Bomb* a dud, but today's dire warnings are predicting the direct opposite catastrophe. In June 2023, *The Economist*[27] declared "Global fertility has collapsed, with profound economic consequences." Likewise, the United Nations[28], which had warned against alarmism in the years following Ehrlich's book tour, admits that "fears of an 'underpopulation crisis' are rising," even though "the world's population has more than doubled in just 50 years, and the global fertility rate remains above the so-

26 *https://www.smithsonianmag.com/innovation/book-incited-worldwide-fear-overpopulation-180967499/*

27 *https://www.economist.com/leaders/2023/06/01/global-fertility-has-collapsed-with-profound-economic-consequences*

28 *https://www.unfpa.org/swp2023/too-few*

called 'replacement-level' of 2.1 births per woman." The anxiety comes from data showing that "an estimated two thirds of the world population [are] now living in a country or area with sub-replacement fertility."

Ironically, the most economically secure nations are the ones with declining birthrates. Europe is facing a population decrease of seven percent between now and 2050. In other developed countries that experience population increases, the driving force may not be births, but immigration.

Are we facing a dystopian future where humans will find it harder to reproduce? This was the scenario in the 1992 novel *Children of Men* by P.D. James. Set in 2021, the book describes a world where no woman has given birth anywhere for almost 20 years. Ms. James never reveals the mysterious cause of global infertility, but the issue in her book lies with the men, who are not producing viable sperm. Certainly, there are environmental factors that can and do affect fertility in men and women, but despite toxicity in the air, food, and water, this imaginative piece of fiction has little basis in fact.

Our world is not so much facing an organic fertility crisis as a birth-rate downturn due to lifestyle choices. Women in Europe and North America don't seem to be any less able to conceive than they have been in previous decades. However, women in developed nations, who have economic opportunities outside of marriage, are delaying marriage and motherhood. For many, this means trying to conceive in their mid-thirties, which is the tail end of their reproductive viability. For some, the fact that they have used prescription birth control for an extended period can also interfere with conception. Their partners are also older, which is a further complication.

I hope this does not sound insensitive towards women who have arrived at a time in their life when they want to be mothers and find themselves unable to get pregnant. But human physiology is what it is. According to the American College of Obstetricians and Gynecologists[29], "A woman's peak reproductive years are between the late teens and late 20s. By age 30, fertility (the ability to get pregnant) starts to decline. This decline happens faster once you reach your mid-30s. By 45, fertility has declined so much that getting pregnant naturally is unlikely." For men also, fertility declines with age. The difference is that even older men will continue to produce sperm, while women have a finite supply of eggs. If man and woman are both in their late 30s, conception is not as easy as it would be if they were both in their 20s.

Infertility, no matter the cause, is a painful reality for many people. According to the World Health Organization[30], "Around 17.5 percent of the adult population—roughly 1 in 6 worldwide—experience infertility." Many couples turn to fertility specialists, who provide in vitro fertilization services for about $15,000 to $20,000 a cycle. A 2011 study[31] found that the average cost for successful IVF treatment ran to $61,377. This makes the process prohibitively expensive for the vast majority of couples.

29 *https://www.acog.org/womens-health/faqs/having-a-baby-after-age-35-how-aging-affects-fertility-and-pregnancy*

30 *https://www.who.int/news/item/04-04-2023-1-in-6-people-globally-affected-by-infertility*

31 *https://www.ncbi.nlm.nih.gov/pmc/articles/PMC3043157/*

Fortunately, NAD may offer a solution for this problem as well. A recent article in *iScience*[32] reports on research which suggests that NAD+ optimization might address age-related decline in female fertility. The authors of the study note that "The ovary is a dynamic organ consisting of heterogeneous cell types that must function coordinately to enable female reproductive function." So, right away, recalling NAD's role in cell signaling, we can expect our favorite molecule to serve an important purpose.

The authors note that mammals have a limited, non-renewable reserve of ovarian follicles, which form very early in the creature's development. These follicles are small sacs filled with fluid. Beginning at puberty, these follicles secrete hormones, which regulate the menstrual cycle. Women begin puberty with about 300,000 to 400,000 follicles, each of which has the potential to release an egg for fertilization. "The ovarian reserve undergoes a natural winnowing over time combined with diminished egg quality, which together contribute to decreased fertility in females by their late 30s and eventual complete cessation of reproductive function at menopause." Thus, women have a limited reproductive lifespan.

By now, it should not surprise us to find that NAD+ assists in ovary function. These cells require energy, and NAD+ acts as a "cofactor, co-substrate, and redox partner in important metabolic pathways involved in energy generation, cell signaling, and tissue repair." Thus, "NAD+ regulates energy metabolism in several ovarian cells." Ovulation, the phase of the menstrual cycle when an egg (ovum) is released from an ovary, requires

32 *https://www.sciencedirect.com/science/article/pii/S2589004223020266*

a great deal of NAD+ "to support follicular rupture, cumulus-oocyte complex release, and corpus luteum formation." NAD+ is also highly necessary for "DNA damage repair which is critical for the prevention of chromosomal abnormalities and maintenance of genetic integrity." Chromosomal abnormalities, or aberrations, manifest in children as Down syndrome, Turner syndrome, trisomy 18 and trisomy 13, as well as a variety of birth defects, dysmorphic facial features, and delays in growth and development. Doctors have long recognized maternal age as a factor in chromosomal abnormalities.

Given "the central role of NAD+ in mediating ovarian metabolism and…function," we should not be surprised to find "a strong association between decline in ovarian NAD+ levels and loss of ovarian function." This decline comes when the demand for NAD+ increases "under survival circumstances, such as the constant need for DNA repair caused by cumulative oxidative stress." Just as NAD+ levels in other organs decline with age, NAD+ levels in the ovaries subside, as women also experience "a decrease in [egg] quantity and quality."

To test the efficacy of NAD+ optimization in assisting female fertility, the researchers took mice that were aging out of their reproductive lifespan and supplemented their diet with NAD+ precursors. The researchers found that "Supplementation with NAD+ precursors, such as nicotinamide mononucleotide (NMN) or nicotinamide riboside (NR), increase NAD+ levels and improve gamete quality, ovarian function, and fertility in aged mice."

The study notes that the glycoprotein CD38 seems to play a role in "age-associated cellular dysfunction" in various tissues throughout the body, including the ovaries. Cellular CD38 increases with age, as NAD+ diminishes. The researchers assert that "CD38 is a negative regulator of reproductive function in reproductively adult females." In other words, this glycoprotein works to shut down female fertility. It would seem that NAD+ optimization arrests the CD38, thereby extending the female's reproductive lifespan.

Since NAD+ is integrally involved in more than 500 cellular processes in the human body, it should not surprise us to find that low levels of NAD+ contribute to infertility. If you or someone you love is struggling with infertility, this new evidence should give them great hope.

Sleep Disorders and Chronic Fatigue

Persistent exhaustion is truly a condition of our time. Wherever I go, I'm confronted by people who complain they are "dead tired" all the time. Many understand this is a consequence of poor sleep, but their efforts to improve their "sleep hygiene," i.e., methods of controlling the behavior and environment related to sleep, have not yielded results. They still suffer from persistent insomnia which robs them of energy, dampens their mood, raises their stress level, and worsens a host of metabolic conditions. It is unfortunate that for so many people, the secret to a good night's sleep remains shrouded in mystery.

INSOMNIA — We all know that a poor night's sleep leaves us cranky and interferes with our day. But chronic poor sleep also makes the body vulnerable to disease. Often, chronic poor sleep is due to problems in the circadian rhythm, a natural oscillation that occurs within organisms on roughly a 24-hour basis. A healthy circadian rhythm tells you when to sleep and when to wake. Disruptions in this sleep-wake cycle have been linked to imbalances in genes and molecules. In other words, to problems on the cellular level. These imbalances are also associated with age-related diseases that include cancer, diabetes, and high blood pressure.

In studies of mice[33] that lack a gene of the sleep-wake cycle, researchers have found that numerous age-related disorders are present. In humans, too, studies have linked metabolic disorders like obesity, insulin resistance, cardiovascular disease, and cancer to abnormalities in the sleep-wake cycle. Researchers have found that NAD+ levels oscillate during the sleep-wake cycle. When NAD+ levels are depleted, either due to age or other factors, the circadian rhythm does not function as well as it should. Thus, optimizing NAD+ levels should reset the circadian rhythm and help restore normal sleep patterns and stave off many age-related diseases.

In 2022, researchers in Japan[34] published a randomized, double-blind placebo-controlled study, which found that a 12-week supplement of the NAD precursor nicotinamide mononucleotide (NMN) each afternoon helped older adults improve the quality of their sleep, reduce drowsiness, and improve lower limb function. Researchers noted that these improvements could "benefit their physical and mental health." Researchers are now pursuing the question of whether oral supplementation of NMN can treat chronic insomnia.

Among our clients, we have much anecdotal evidence that our NAD supplementation delivers deeper, more restorative sleep for individuals who have struggled with insomnia. This

33 *https://www.nmn.com/news/nad-and-the-sleep-wake-cycle*

34 *https://www.ncbi.nlm.nih.gov/pmc/articles/PMC8877443/*

is great news for their overall health, because as it is often said, "Sleep is medicine." When we sleep well, we can enjoy good health and deter a wide range of illnesses.

CHRONIC FATIGUE SYNDROME — It would seem that, for people who simply can't get to sleep or stay asleep, NAD delivers strong benefits. But there are also people who suffer from chronic fatigue syndrome, or myalgic encephalomyelitis, a complicated disorder consisting of many symptoms with no obvious cause. Symptoms vary from patient to patient, and their severity fluctuates from day to day. The unifying theme is extreme fatigue that lasts for at least six months, during which the patient can also experience:

- Problems with memory or cognitive skills
- Dizziness upon sitting or standing from a prone position
- Muscle or joint pain

Perhaps the most frustrating aspect of this syndrome is that these patients can sleep for long periods, but their sleep does not refresh them. They can awaken after a full night of sleep and the first thing they crave is a nap. Many patients also suffer from headaches, sore throats, and tender lymph nodes in the neck or armpits. They may become acutely sensitive to light, sound, smells, food, and medicines.

Chronic fatigue syndrome often worsens under stress, making it extremely difficult to maintain employment and relationships, so patients see the scope of their lives narrow until there's little left but sleeping and waking.

So, what could cause such a debilitating condition? Although the exact cause is still unknown, experts cite a combination of four factors that may contribute:

- **GENETICS** — Chronic fatigue syndrome appears to run in some families, so some people may be born with a higher likelihood of developing the disorder. However, we must also consider lifestyle habits, because families often share these important determinants of health. It's the age-old question of nature versus nurture.
- **INFECTIONS** — Some patients develop symptoms after recovering from a viral or bacterial infection. That raises the question of whether the infection has totally cleared from their system or might be persisting at a lower level.
- **PHYSICAL OR EMOTIONAL TRAUMA** — Some patients recall experiencing an accidental injury, surgery, or significant emotional stress prior to the emergence of their symptoms.
- **METABOLIC PROBLEMS** — Some chronic fatigue patients have trouble with energy usage due to their body's inability to convert fats and sugars into energy.

It's worth noting that additional risk factors exist, including:

- **AGE** — Although chronic fatigue syndrome can occur at any time, young-to-middle-aged adults are most commonly affected.
- **SEX** — Women receive the lion's share of CFS diagnoses, but practitioners caution us from drawing too firm a conclusion on this point. It could be that men are simply less likely to report their condition and are suffering with CFS in silence.

- **RELATED MEDICAL PROBLEMS** — Patients with a history of certain medical problems, such as fibromyalgia or postural orthostatic tachycardia syndrome, seem more likely to develop CFS.

Chronic fatigue syndrome is a complex puzzle for medical minds, and I am not going to suggest that NAD is a magic bullet. More study is certainly needed. However, we know that NAD helps the body manufacture energy on the cellular level. That undisputable fact is cause for optimism.

One area of scientific inquiry worth noting is the relationship between tryptophan metabolism and certain physical and psychological symptoms often found in CFS. Tryptophan is an essential amino acid that infants need for normal growth and which all humans rely on for the production and maintenance of the body's proteins, muscles, enzymes, and neurotransmitters. You might know tryptophan as the compound that makes you drowsy after a big turkey dinner. It is widely used as a sleep regulator and to help muscle recovery after strenuous workouts. But to be of any help, the body must metabolize the tryptophan on the cellular level, often via the kynurenine pathway (KP).

Abnormalities in the kynurenine pathway[35] have been observed in patients with major depressive disorder. MDD is a condition characterized by persistently low or depressed mood, decreased interest in pleasurable activities, feelings of guilt or worthlessness, lack of energy, poor concentration, appetite changes, agitation, sleep disturbances, or suicidal

35 *https://www.sciencedirect.com/topics/biochemistry-genetics-and-molecular-biology/kynurenine-pathway*

thoughts. Problems with the kynurenine pathway have been noted in patients with bi-polar depression. These observations have led researchers to ask whether KP problems could not also contribute to CFS.

A July 11, 2022, article in the journal *Cellular and Molecular Life Sciences*[36] is entitled, *Could the kynurenine pathway be the key missing piece of Myalgic Encephalomyelitis/Chronic Fatigue Syndrome (ME/CFS) complex puzzle?* The authors state that the kynurenine pathway "has been shown to mediate immune response and neuroinflammation," which are functions impaired in patients with CFS. The authors assert that certain "KP abnormalities and symptoms…are classic characteristics of ME/CFS."

But what does KP have to do with NAD? According to this article, the kynurenine pathway "plays a central role in cellular energy production through the production of nicotinamide adenine dinucleotide (NADH)." NADH is very closely related to NAD+, the only difference being a hydrogen atom with an extra electron. The article's authors assert that "KP regulation may provide innovative approaches to the management of ME/CFS." It is therefore possible that NAD+ or a related molecule could hold the key to alleviating symptoms of CFS.

Of course, not every case of fatigue, no matter how regularly it occurs, fits the definition of chronic fatigue syndrome. How many of us suffer from horrendous afternoon slumps? Yours might come immediately after eating lunch, no matter how light a meal you take. Or at the stroke of three pm, you might think, "I have to nap or die." In these cases, NAD+

36 https://pubmed.ncbi.nlm.nih.gov/35821534/

might be just the tonic. Here's how Dr. James Goodwin, author of *Supercharge Your Brain*, describes his experience:

> *"Over the last year, I started experiencing really debilitating fatigue in the afternoon. About six months ago, I did the NAD test and got shockingly low results coming in deficient. I'm perfectly healthy. I don't have any diagnosed medical conditions. I exercise regularly, I eat well, and I'm not overweight.*
>
> *"I was so appalled and determined to start taking the supplements regularly.*
>
> *"Two weeks into taking the NAD supplement, the fatigue disappeared. I was absolutely astonished. I'm not going to stop taking the supplements to see if the fatigue comes back. I'd recommend the* Vitality Boost *to anyone who needs extra energy."*

If *Vitality Boost* gets the nod from this medical authority, maybe it can help you from nodding off in the middle of the day.

Cancer

There is perhaps no more terrifying medical diagnosis than cancer, especially in the late stages. In decades past, a cancer diagnosis was a death sentence. Fortunately, medical science has advanced to the point where survival rates from many cancers are encouraging. But many therapies to become "cancer free" are still excruciating and subject the patient to debilitating side effects. Thus, it's important to understand cancer risks and modify our lifestyle to reduce the likelihood of cancer, and to follow protocols that enable early detection, so the disease is more treatable.

But what exactly is cancer? And how does it start? Most people understand that cancer is a mutation of the cells from normal, healthy building blocks to an invasive and hostile force. We call cancer cells "malignant," which means "tending to produce death or deterioration." Additionally, we understand that these malignant cells form clusters we call tumors, which displace healthy tissues, multiplying more aggressively that the healthy tissue, until the healthy tissues can no longer support the afflicted body part, causing a cascading failure of function that culminates in death.

It is worth noting that risk factors for cancer overlap significantly with other illnesses and metabolic disorders, such as cardiovascular disease, insulin resistance, and type II diabetes. According to World Health Organization, common risk factors for cancer include:

- Tobacco use
- Alcohol use
- Overweight and obesity
- Dietary factors, including insufficient fruit and vegetable intake
- Physical inactivity

Other factors to consider include chronic infections and environmental risks, such as radiation.

But to truly understand cancer, we must know what is happening at the cellular level. Our cells are constantly reproducing through the process of mitosis, during which a cell duplicates all of its contents, including its chromosomes, and splits to form two identical cells. For reasons not fully understood, mitosis can go wrong, producing cells with damaged DNA. These mutated cells can continue to replicate, forming malignant tumors.

From decades of studying cancer, we know that these mutations are more likely to occur in older individuals. There is even a fatalistic attitude in medical circles that any individual who lives long enough will contract cancer. Thus, even though many children suffer the scourge of juvenile cancer, the condition is predominantly a disease of mature age.

This forces us to consider what is happening to human cells as we age. From my study of age-related illnesses, I know that the molecular makeup of human cells is different in older individuals compared to those who are significantly younger. One noteworthy difference is that older people have lower levels of intracellular NAD+. And, since NAD+ is necessary for producing the energy that enables cellular functions, including mitosis, it is logical to wonder whether lower levels of NAD+ impede mitosis, or allow DNA to be damaged in the process. It is not unreasonable to suppose that maintaining healthy, youthful NAD+ levels into mature adulthood can forestall cancer.

The situation may be different, however, for individuals who already have cancer. NAD+ is an essential molecule for intracellular energy and cell division even in cancer cells. This means that cancer cells might be hungry for NAD and might use it to supercharge tumor growth. Thus, researchers are exploring how best to manage NAD+ levels in cancer patients. Some cancer scientists believe that lowering NAD+ levels could be a key to slowing tumor growth, while others believe that combining conventional anti-cancer treatments with

NAD+ supplementation will target malignant cells while improving the overall health of the patient.

In an article entitled, *The Key Role of NAD+ in Anti-Tumor Immune Response: An Update*, published in the journal *Frontiers in Immunology* in April 2021[37], researchers argue that NAD+ supplementation can boost the activity of T cells, those white blood cells that fight infection as part of the body's immune response. T cells see cancer as "foreign" cells that don't belong, so they attack and try to destroy the cancerous cells. However, T cells are often suppressed by CD38, a multifunctional protein that seems to work beneficially when NAD+ levels are healthy but accelerates aging and suppresses the immune system when NAD+ is depleted.

Earlier in this book, we discussed how NAD+ seems to keep CD38 expression in check. The *FII* article notes that CD38 inhibits "anti-tumor immune response ... in solid and hematological tumors." In other words, too much active CD38 can prevent T cells from seeking and destroying cancer cells. This effect has been observed in chronic lymphocytic leukemia. Is it possible that NAD+ optimization can stifle CD38's suppressive activity, freeing the T cells to defend the body? This would be a game changer for cancer patients, because it would empower their own immune system to fight off cancer, rather than relying on harsh therapies that also take a heavy toll on healthy tissues.

This is an area of inquiry I would like to see pursued. Imagine if we could gather data on the intracellular NAD levels of

37 *https://www.frontiersin.org/articles/10.3389/fimmu.2021.658263/full*

patients recently diagnosed with cancer. Would we see a correlation between low NAD levels and cancer? But we must also try to gather data from healthy individuals, such as those who live into their 70s and 80s without developing cancer. There is so much we can learn from their biomarkers that could help in the prevention and treatment of disease. Armed with this information, we could help countless people enjoy an extended healthspan.

Healthy Vision

We all know that vision declines with age. As we grow older, we all become far-sighted, meaning that we have difficulty seeing objects up close. This condition is called presbyopia, which literally means "the vision of the elder." Thus, it makes sense that if we can slow the aging process through NAD optimization, we can maintain healthy vision longer. But researchers have also found that NAD may help address a severe threat to eyesight for which there is currently no cure.

AGE-RELATED MACULAR DEGENERATION — Imagine going blind in the prime of your life. You've had no symptoms of disease, but suddenly your central vision is blurry or wavy. In time, you can see nothing that's right in front of you, though you can see objects clearly with your peripheral vision. That is the situation for an alarming number of American adults. The cause is age-related macular degeneration (AMD), which is a leading cause of vision loss for Americans ages 50 and older.

A study published in *JAMA Ophthalmology*, entitled, *The Prevalence of Age-Related Macular Degeneration in the United*

States In 2019[38], found that 19.83 million Americans were living with some form of age-related macular degeneration. The lion's share of those diagnosed, estimated at 18.34 million, had early AMD, which often goes undetected and untreated. However, 1.49 million had the late-stage, vision-threatening form of AMD, for which there is no effective treatment. To put this in perspective, approximately one in 10 Americans ages 50 and older have early AMD, and approximately one of every 100 Americans aged 50 and older have the late form. Although most will not lose their vision until their 70s, loss of vision at any age severely undermines a person's quality of life. Loss of sight means loss of independence. Imagine working all your life to retire and enjoy your favorite activities, perhaps do a little traveling to see parts of the world you've never experienced, and suddenly you've lost your most vital sense. When we talk about optimum healthspan, we want to do all we can to deter diseases like AMD.

Avoidance is key, because there is currently no cure for AMD. The best that medical science can offer at the moment is advice on lifestyle modification to slow the progression. What do ophthalmologists recommend for patients diagnosed with early AMD? Stop me if you've heard this before:

- Adopt a healthy diet
- Stop smoking
- Supplement antioxidants
- Address high blood pressure

38 *https://jamanetwork.com/journals/jamaophthalmology/fullarticle/2797921*

If you're thinking that these steps are applicable to a wide range of metabolic disorders that worsen with age, bravo! You're seeing the pattern. If you also noted that these are corrective measures for oxidative stress, which can cause mitochondrial dysfunction, leading to DNA damage, you know where I'm going. If NAD has proven useful for correcting other age-related illnesses, particularly those related to oxidative stress, why couldn't NAD+ help with AMD? There is good reason to believe it can, but first, let's take a closer look at the disease.

There are two primary types of AMD, which have different causes:

- **DRY AMD** is by far the most common, afflicting about 80 percent of patients. While its exact cause is unknown, researchers suspect that genetic and environmental factors play a role. Patients lose vision because the light-sensitive cells in the macula—the part of the retina at the back of the eye, which controls central vision—slowly break down, usually one eye at a time. Vision loss is usually slow and gradual. By now, when I mention cells breaking down, you're probably thinking that age-related NAD+ depletion is contributing to problems for healthy cell replication. So, hold that thought.
- **WET AMD** is less common and usually leads to more severe vision loss. Wet AMD occurs when abnormal blood vessels start to grow beneath the retina. These cells leak fluid and blood—hence the term "wet" AMD—and can create a large blind spot in the center of the visual field. Again, you might wonder why there is abnormal cell growth. Has something happened to the intracellular environment to damage DNA? Did the process of healthy cell replication break down because an essential

component was missing? Might that component be NAD?

A 2019 study, published in the journal *Discovery Medicine*[39], entitled, *NAD+ Inhibits the Metabolic Reprogramming of RPE Cells in Early Age-related Macular Degeneration by Upregulating Mitophagy* states that "NAD+ has proven benefits as a central metabolic cofactor in the eye. Future studies evaluating NAD+ metabolism in the context of aging and AMD development and progression are highly warranted."

More recently, the journal *Mechanisms of Aging and Development*[40] published a study in January 2023, entitled, *The role of NAD+ metabolism in macrophages in age-related macular degeneration.* The authors of this report found evidence that "decreased intracellular NAD+ levels and overexpression of CD38" are possible factors in AMD. You'll recall that we've already discussed the benefits of NAD+ counteracting CD38 in female infertility and cancer. If CD38 is a factor in AMD, it's logical to think that NAD+ could alleviate the condition or at least slow its progression.

While these studies are by no means definitive, they strongly suggest that NAD+ supplementation should be part of the preventative regimen for patients diagnosed with AMD. Antioxidant supplements alone cannot stop AMD in its tracks. Bolstered by NAD+, these compounds have a greater chance

39 *https://www.discoverymedicine.com/Qingquan-Wei-2/2019/05/nad-inhibits-reprogramming-of-rpe-cells-in-early-amd-by-upregulating-mitophagy/*

40 *https://www.sciencedirect.com/science/article/abs/pii/S0047637422001373*

of correcting the mitochondrial issues that lead to the abnormal cell growth that causes vision loss.

Allergies and Asthma

Countless people are tormented by allergies. Their eyes water, their noses run, they sneeze, their skin breaks out in hives, and in extreme cases they can go into shock. Why do their bodies react so violently to substances that are generally benign? Why do some people have allergies while others do not? These are questions which medical science has not adequately answered.

What we do know is that allergies are an immune system reaction that releases antibodies to combat a substance identified as a threat. Unfortunately, the reaction is far worse than any harm the triggering substance could cause if it were simply left alone. In the worst-case scenario, an allergy sufferer can experience anaphylaxis, a life-threatening medical emergency, characterized by some or all of the following symptoms:

- Loss of consciousness
- A drop in blood pressure
- Severe shortness of breath
- Skin rash
- Lightheadedness
- A rapid, weak pulse
- Nausea and vomiting

Many allergy sufferers also must deal with asthma, an immune system reaction that affects the airways and breathing. According to the Cleveland Clinic, about 25 million Americans suffer from asthma, and 60 percent of those cases are related to allergies. Asthma can prevent a person from exhaling, so they cannot refill their lungs with fresh air, leading to asphyxia. Allergies and asthma often react to the same environmental stimuli. But what is it that makes the body wrongly identify certain particles, such as dust or pollen, as deadly enemies?

First, we should note that allergies and asthma have a genetic component[41]. It's been apparent for a long time that asthma runs in families and that children of asthmatic parents are at increased risk of asthma. But the transmission of this disease is not as straightforward as other inherited traits, such as eye color, or classic monogenic diseases, such as Huntington's disease or sickle-cell disease. Those conditions rely on the mutation of a single gene. Asthma, on the other hand, is a polygenic, multifactorial disorder. Some studies suggest there are as many as 100 genes[42] and combinations thereof at play, as well as environmental factors, which contribute to making a person asthmatic. This makes asthma similar to autism. Many individuals may have a gene combination that makes them susceptible to the illness, but they must also be exposed to outside forces that trigger the condition.

Some medical professionals also believe there is an emotional/psychological link with allergies and asthma. To understand this thinking, we might look at the life of America's most famous asthma sufferer: Theodore Roosevelt. By all accounts, this child of a wealthy family had an idyllic childhood, but a sinister tension lurked beneath the surface of his privileged family. His father was a Yankee from New York, and his

41 *https://www.ncbi.nlm.nih.gov/pmc/articles/PMC4629762/*

42 *https://medlineplus.gov/genetics/condition/allergic-asthma*

mother was a daughter of the Confederacy. Early in Teddy's childhood, those regions were embroiled in a bloody war. As Southern fortunes turned from bad to worse, news of the war took a terrible toll on Teddy's mother, and he would often experience violent attacks of asthma. His parents treated Teddy's spells by making him drink strong coffee and take a few puffs from his father's cigar. (We should be grateful that even though modern medicine hasn't cured asthma, it has at least advanced far enough to give us the rescue inhaler!)

As young Roosevelt grew, he was gaunt and spindly. But, determined to develop his sickly frame, he took up boxing at Harvard. He even traveled out West to work as a cowboy, thinking the outdoors would deliver a cure. Roosevelt succeeded in building himself into a robust "Rough Rider," and for a time was seen as the epitome of the energy behind American progress. Ultimately, his lungs betrayed him, as he passed away from a pulmonary embolism at age 60.

In Roosevelt, we see the possibility of a genetic predisposition towards asthma activated from chronic nervousness in childhood. Certainly, a pervasive feeling of dread, related to his mother's anxiety about the war, could have caused hypersensitivity in his immune system. By sheer willpower, he surmounted that obstacle to become an accomplished statesman, but he never really left his childhood affliction behind. Building up his musculature was a great tonic (as we shall see in the next section), but it was not sufficient to work a cure.

Teddy Roosevelt is fairly typical of asthmatic boys whose symptoms are extreme in childhood but become milder with age. However, asthma is also an "adult onset" disease, occurring in people aged 20 and older. The majority of these sufferers are women, and researchers believe this could be due to hormonal changes. Some adult-onset cases are due to viral or bacterial infections, or the cumulative effects of irritants, ranging from tobacco smoke to industrial chemicals.

Caustic substances in the environment can give rise to a condition called industrial asthma. Factory workers and miners have historically been vulnerable to breathing problems due to harsh chemicals in the workplace and toxic dust in the mines. We've also seen a large number of rescue workers at Ground Zero of the 9/11 terrorist attack develop asthma due to the smoldering cauldron of toxic rubble. Exposure to toxins can make a person more vulnerable to minor irritants, such as dust and pollen, so that asthma attacks become more frequent and intense.

Today there is still no cure for allergies or allergic asthma, but recent research suggests that NAD precursor supplementation can ease symptoms. For example, an article entitled, *Nicotinamide mononucleotide attenuates airway epithelial barrier dysfunction via inhibiting SIRT3 SUMOylation in asthma*, was published in the journal *International Immunopharmacology* for January 25, 2024.[43] The conclusion is fairly well captured in the title. This study demonstrated that "restoring cellular NAD+ concentration through supplementation" in asthmatic mice "alleviated airway inflammation and reduced mucus secretion." Supplementation also "mitigated airway … disruption." However, the study also showed that inhibition of SIRT3, a mitochondrial sirtuin, which usually works in conjunction

43 *https://www.sciencedirect.com/science/article/abs/pii/S1567576923016557*

with NAD to promote cellular homeostasis, obliterated the positive effects of NAD precursor supplementation.

Of course, the deadliest type of allergic/asthmatic reaction is anaphylaxis, characterized by a severe airway constriction that can easily cause asphyxiation. Anaphylaxis can also include hives, swelling, low blood pressure, abdominal pain, and severe diarrhea. These symptoms are due to a process which scientists call Mast Cell Activation. Mast cells are a type of white blood cell found in connective tissues throughout the body, especially under the skin, near blood vessels and lymph vessels, in nerves, and in the lungs and intestines. Mast cells secrete different chemicals during allergic reactions. In Mast Cell Activation, these key immune defenders go haywire, overreacting to the perceived threat to the body. Mast Cell Activation Syndrome, where a patient suffers repeat episodes of this phenomenon, is a potentially grave allergic disorder.

Scientists have studied mast cell signaling to improve our understanding of the pathophysiology of anaphylaxis to develop novel approaches to treatment. A recent study was published in April of 2022 in the journal *Theranostics*.[44] The researchers noted that the role of NAD+ "in mast cell function, especially in response to an anaphylactic condition, has remained unexplored." The researchers looked at whether optimizing NAD+ levels through precursor supplementation would prevent "mast cell degranulation and anaphylactic responses." They found that "NAD+-boosting molecules" do "suppress mast cell degranulation and anaphylactic responses in mice." Therefore, "NAD+ precursors may serve as an effective therapeutic strategy that limits mast cell-mediated anaphylactic responses." In

44 *https://www.ncbi.nlm.nih.gov/pmc/articles/PMC9065190/*

other words, NAD optimization may prevent the worst kind of allergic reactions.

Allergies and asthma are a complicated puzzle, and research focused on intracellular processes is still in its infancy. Yet, early signs point to NAD as an important piece in any eventual solution. I believe we can be confident that NAD+ will prove efficacious for the following reasons:

- **REGULATION OF IMMUNE CELLS** — NAD influences the function and regulation of various immune cells, including T cells, B cells, and macrophages. By fine tuning the activity of these cells, NAD can potentially alter the immune system's reactivity to allergens, offering a new avenue for allergy management.
- **REDUCTION OF INFLAMMATORY RESPONSE** — Inflammation is a hallmark of allergic reactions, manifesting as redness, swelling, and discomfort. NAD plays a role in the signaling pathways that regulate inflammation. By influencing these pathways, NAD can potentially modulate the body's inflammatory response to allergens, leading to a reduction in the severity of symptoms, so that pollen season becomes more bearable.
- **REGULATION OF SIRTUIN ACTIVITY** — we've said a lot already about these NAD-dependent enzymes which are instrumental for cellular health, longevity, and stress resistance. Sirtuins also play a crucial part in regulating inflammation and immune responses. Activation of sirtuins could help mitigate the inflammatory processes associated with allergic reactions. But that activation depends heavily on optimal levels of NAD+.

- **NAD PRECURSORS SUPPRESS HYPERALLERGIC REACTIONS** — As we mention above, researchers have found that one of the building blocks of NAD+, nicotinamide, inhibits the release of pro-inflammatory proteins called histamines from white blood cells called mast cells. Mast cell histamine release is a hallmark of the life-threatening anaphylactic response. If NAD+ precursors can alleviate the worst-case allergic response, there's every reason to hope they can assist with common allergies.

Also giving reason for hope are the individual testimonials we get from *Jinfiniti* clients who discover that allergy relief is an unexpected bonus. First, there is Jimmy, 65 years old, who is the floor manager at a high-end steakhouse. This is a customer-facing position, where you wouldn't want to appear with watery eyes and a runny nose. But Jimmy had severe allergies with sneezing and nasal congestion, and even on prescription meds, he went through a box of tissues a day. In addition, Jimmy has atrial fibrillation and high blood pressure, so he can't take OTC decongestants. Therefore, he was paying a high price for drugs without getting much benefit. Like many allergy sufferers, Jimmy found his condition was getting progressively worse with age. No longer seasonal, his allergies haunted him year 'round.

Then, Jimmy found *Vitality Boost*. After about eight months, Jimmy told us his symptoms had lessened considerably. But not only did his allergies improve, his blood pressure became more manageable as well. He also said he has more stamina on the job. That's an important bonus since Jimmy's restaurant job requires him to spend long hours on his feet as he covers about six-to-eight walking miles a day.

Next up is Emily, who left this message on our website in January of 2024:

> *"I originally bought this supplement for its longevity support, but to my surprise, it helped with my allergies! We have a dog who sadly gives me lots of sneezing fits, stuffy noses, and occasional asthmatic reactions.*
>
> *"I have taken everything under the sun that the doctor has prescribed. Some of those things have helped mildly, others not so much, but I know every pharmaceutical comes with a cost. I am happy to say I am now able to nix the daily* Zyrtec *that was previously needed to cope after a month of using* Vitality *and am using only Singulair and my emergency inhaler.*
>
> *"Next up, I will try to ease out of a* Singulair. *Wish me luck!"*

We wish Emily, Jimmy, and every other allergy sufferer all the luck in the world.

Strength and Stamina

We can all use a little more strength and stamina, but no one craves this enhancement more than professional athletes hoping to make their marks in their respective sports. For many of these hopefuls, NAD+ optimization has become a routine part of their training regimen. Unfortunately, some are acting upon misinformation and are using costly methods that provide little benefit. One such athlete was pro boxer Sena Agebeko, the current WBC Super Middle Weight Champion.

When we met him, Sena had already been supplementing NAD intravenously. He reports, "When I was first told about

Jinfiniti, I had my doubts. I believed a lot in NAD IV." However, after taking our biomarker test, he found that those expensive and inconvenient IVs had not optimized his intracellular NAD. His level was only at 20! But in two weeks of using *Vitality Boost*, his NAD+ more than tripled to a robust 65.

"I noticed my training improved," Sena told us. "My stamina in my workouts was much greater. I was running longer, faster, and my strength levels were up. Plus, I battle anxiety and it's been much better…and I won my next fight in two rounds which felt easy."

Sena's results are not isolated. Track star Celera Barnes is another celebrity *Jinfiniti* client. Celera has run track since age 11, and in high school she won the 200-meter dash at the California high school championships. She went on to star for UCLA, University of Kentucky, and USC, earning three degrees before exhausting her NCAA eligibility. She was a member of the World Championship relay team in 2022. Celera signed an endorsement deal with Adidas and is now in her second year of professional track, training for the 2024 Summer Olympics in Paris.

Celera had been taking supplements to boost her NAD+ for about five years, which she credited with increasing her energy and boosting her performance. Then her high school coach recommended she switch to *Jinfiniti*'s *Vitality Boost* in October 2023. Right away she noticed she had more energy. She felt much stronger and recovered more quickly after strenuous workouts. Although she didn't have her NAD+ levels tested, Celera believes that *Vitality Boost* delivered "a higher degree of benefits."

She has since made the first USA world team as an individual, finishing in the top three in the country for the indoor 60-meter dash. When we spoke to her, she was excited about the Olympic trials, set for June 21, 2024, in Eugene, Oregon.

Speaking of running, here is what one long-distance runner has to say about *Vitality Boost*:

> *"I recently purchased the* Vitality Boost *in October of 2023 and have used it since...I didn't know that it could increase energy and improve performance, and being in the military while on deployment has given me that extra boost to get me through my long days.*
>
> *"...This product couldn't have come at a better time since I was preparing for the Athens Marathon in Greece on November 12th, 2023. I finished 608th of 21,598, averaging a pace of 7:30 seconds for a distance of 26.2 miles. For proof, check out my Instagram @ _mas_oficial, which shows my race results! This was my first marathon, and being a 31-year-old male, I felt like I was in my early 20s. I feel more energized and focused throughout the day while in the field."*
>
> *—Emmanuel C.*

And for those who want to walk before they can run:

> *"Within two weeks of taking the* Vitality Boost *I noticed my energy levels increasing. Additionally, I have always been a walker, but this past summer I was often fatigued after 3 or 4 miles. After taking it for a month or so, I'd walk 10-15 miles without fatigue."*
>
> *—Dawn.*

There is no doubt that NAD+ optimization improves stamina, especially in older adults, as this client testifies:

> *"I have used other NAD products but at 75 years old, I was still testing just low normal, and not feeling able to complete my normal day and workouts with vigor. After six weeks using* Jinfiniti's Vitality Boost *I am back living like I was 25 years ago... Five-to-10-mile hikes, full days of meetings and studying... and having fun again! My wife is also back to our expected normal activity levels..."*
>
> *—Bruce Ross*

Those of us who are not professional athletes are fully content with the strength for our routine chores and recreational pastimes. We think that by "bulking up" our muscle mass, we become slaves to our bodies, rather than conditioning our bodies to serve us. But medical science is developing a greater understanding of the long-term benefits of robust muscle mass and, conversely, the detriments to our health when we do not have well-conditioned muscles. Not surprisingly, NAD+ plays a vital role.

MUSCULATURE — Skeletal muscle has been called "the organ of longevity." Individuals who maintain muscle mass into adulthood tend to live longer and healthier lives. Medical professionals have long considered healthy musculature in older adults to be a consequence of good health, but many doctors today believe we've been getting cause and effect backwards, and that sustained good health is a result of well-conditioned muscles.

Dr. Gabrielle Lyon[45] is a strong proponent of building muscles to optimize health and longevity. A functional medicine practitioner and board-certified family medicine physician, Dr. Lyon founded the Institute for Muscle-Centric Medicine. She favors a proactive approach to health over the reactive disease treatment that dominates today's Western medicine. She believes that the key to health lies in "the biggest organ in your body: skeletal muscle." The current population isn't "over(ly) fat." Rather, "we are just under-muscled." She believes our neglect of muscle conditioning "is leading to diseases and chronic aging."

Dr. Lyon asserts there is a link between muscle mass and disease survivability. In humans, both male and female, strength and muscle mass steadily increase from birth to about 30-35 years old. From that point, muscle mass naturally declines with age, a process known as sarcopenia. The decline in muscle power and performance is slow and linear at first, then accelerates after age 65 for women and 70 for men. This is when we often see the onset of age-related illnesses. To slow this process of decline, weight training is essential. But Dr. Lyon contends that exercise which stimulates skeletal muscle not only helps us retain physical strength; such activity also helps us "maintain mobility, mental clarity, hormonal balance, and improve mood."

Dr. Lyon believes that conditioning skeletal muscle "will help you build your body armor to protect you throughout life." That protection continues into old age, making us less prone to debilitating falls and chronic illnesses that lead to premature mortality.

45 *https://worth.com/muscle-is-the-cornerstone-of-longevity/*

Emily Moore, ND, L.Ac[46], a naturopathic doctor at Goshen Center for Cancer Care, agrees with Dr. Lyon. Writing for the website *goshenhealth.com*, Dr. Moore warns that "Less muscle tissue can [negatively] affect your health in several ways." These include:

- Changes metabolism
- Reduces insulin sensitivity
- Increases risk of metabolic diseases, like diabetes, fatty liver, and obesity

Dr. Moore recommends moderate exercise most days of the week along with weight or resistance training twice a week to keep muscles in good shape.

Additional support for muscle conditioning into maturity is found in a 2022 study published in *JAMA Network Open*. According to *The Washington Post*[47], The Canadian Longitudinal Study on Aging found that "the presence of low muscle mass was associated with faster future cognitive function decline in adults at least 65 years old." This might be because "greater muscle mass [results] in more physical activity and cardiorespiratory fitness, which leads to more blood flow to the brain."

Returning to the idea of hormonal balance, briefly mentioned above, we should not that skeletal muscle is the largest *endocrine* organ system in the body. This means that, when active, your muscles secrete hormones and peptides called myokines.

46 *https://goshenhealth.com/blog/is-muscle-the-organ-of-longevity*

47 *https://www.washingtonpost.com/wellness/2023/01/29/strength-training-all-ages/*

Myokines travel throughout the body and interact with the liver and brain and other organs, regulating many other parts of your body from hormonal to immune systems. Thus, your skeletal muscles are great regulators of bodily functions, but they can't do this job if they're underdeveloped, undernourished. and underutilized.

Skeletal muscle is also the place where most of our body's mitochondria resides. Remember, mitochondria are the engines of our cellular energy system. If our skeletal muscle tissue is healthy, those engines will keep humming, enabling every cellular process—such as healing and immunity—to continue in a healthy manner.

Moreover, skeletal muscle is your metabolic disposable unit, used for carbohydrate disposal, fatty acid oxidation, and clearing out bad cholesterol. And, as Dr. Lyon states, skeletal muscle is your body armor. If you get sick, your body will pull reserves of amino acids from your skeletal muscle to combat the disease.

Of course, muscle requires more than exercise to be healthy. Ingesting the proper quantity and quality of protein is imperative since protein is the body's only essential macronutrient. It's also important to have sufficient levels of creatine, a natural compound from three amino acids, which is shown to improve strength, increase lean muscle mass, and help the muscles recover more quickly during exercise.

Within muscle cells, creatine is primarily stored in the form of phosphocreatine, a high-energy compound that serves as a rapid and potent reservoir of phosphate groups. During short bursts of intense physical activity, such as weightlifting or sprinting, phosphocreatine donates its phosphate group to adenosine diphosphate (ADP), regenerating adenosine triphosphate (ATP)—which we know as the primary energy currency of cells. This process enhances the cell's ability to sustain brief, high-intensity efforts. In fact, the primary job of creatine is to replenish ATP. By providing a rapid source of energy, creatine allows individuals to push their physical limits, leading to increased strength, power, and overall athletic performance. It's like having a turbo boost for your muscles.

But creatine's impact extends far beyond the realms of raw muscle strength. Research suggests that it also may have wonderful cognitive benefits, including brain function and potentially aiding tasks that require short bursts of intense mental effort. New research in October 2023 indicates that creatine is also a valuable neurotransmitter that helps to optimize brain function (blog link here w/citation).

Whether you're an elite athlete who is striving for peak performance, a casual gym-goer looking to maximize your workouts, or someone interested in maximizing your brain potential, creatine can be a game-changer. If you're serious about optimizing your physical and mental capabilities, creatine deserves a prime spot in your supplement arsenal. Naturally, *Jinfiniti* has included creatine in our formula for *Vitality Boost*.

Finally, there is the all-important role of NAD in muscular health. You knew we'd get around to this, didn't you? In skeletal muscle, NAD plays a fundamental role in cellular respiration, particularly when it comes to glycolytic and oxidative pathways. During glycolysis, NAD converts certain phosphates into ATP, which, we just noted, is essential for energy during muscle activity.

Creatine and NAD interact in a fascinating dance in the human body. Creatine, the muscle's go-to energy currency, and NAD, the critical coenzyme involved in over 500+ physiological processes, engage in subtle but impactful interplay, because when creatine is replenishing ATP, it requires a small sacrifice of NAD. This exchange might seem like a minor detail, but it highlights the interconnected nature of the two elements.

Some studies even suggest that creatine might have a sparing effect on NAD, potentially helping to maintain its levels during periods of high energy demand. And since NAD is involved in processes like DNA repair and cellular signaling, any influence on its levels could have broader implications beyond just energy metabolism.

In essence, the relationship between creatine and NAD showcases the complexity of our body's biochemical symphony. While each plays a distinct role, their subtle interactions remind us that the pathways governing our physiology are a web of connections, where changes in one component can resonate throughout the entire system—in this case—the human body.

Other compounds that help keep muscles healthy also rely on NAD. NAD-dependent enzymes, such as sirtuins, are involved in various cellular functions, including gene expression, DNA repair, and mitochondrial biogenesis. Sirtuins, activated by NAD, play a vital role in the maintenance of skeletal muscle health by regulating processes like protein synthesis, degradation, and cellular stress responses. NAD has also been implicated in modulating skeletal muscle stem cell function, impacting muscle regeneration and repair.

In essence, it's a circular system. Your body creates more energy with muscular use, and you need energy for that same muscular use. That's why NAD is the missing link, the lifesaving channel for your skeletal muscular system. And this is one of many reasons why testing your NAD levels is vital and supplementing with precursors to boost your NAD levels back to optimal levels is paramount. You cannot derive the longevity benefits from healthy skeletal muscle, if your NAD levels aren't sufficient to produce and maintain healthy skeletal muscle.

CHAPTER 9

MAXIMIZING YOUR HEALTHSPAN THROUGH PRECISION MEDICINE

"To know that there is a limit to what one knows,
This is the truest and highest knowledge."

—Lao-Tzu, *Tao Te Ching*

Lao-Tzu believed that the *Tao* held the key to a long and peaceful life. By refraining from ambitious striving, by living close to nature, and by practicing nonaction to maintain inner peace and our essential unity, we could live longer and enjoy better health. Of course, the desire for a long, healthy life was not unique to ancient China; it has permeated every culture, from the ancients to our present day.

How I'd love to be able to say that, armed with greater scientific knowledge, we are closer than ever to achieving mankind's epic dream of a longer, healthier life. But we all know that greater technical knowledge does not always translate into better lifestyle choices. Especially when nature pleads with us to humbly accept our physical limitations, rather than doing anything we want in the moment.

But scientific knowledge at least gives us a choice. Prior to medical science unlocking the secrets of NAD+, the problems of age-related and metabolic illnesses appeared insurmountable. Some individuals just seemed randomly doomed to poor health. They might try as hard as anyone to improve their condition, but the results didn't come. The persistent question, "Why me?," had no good answer. It's exciting to think that for so many people who care about their health, an answer might finally be available.

I have been a scientist for more than 40 years, but I have never been as excited about what I do on a daily basis as I am today. Our work at *Jinfiniti* is already impacting tens of thousands of people and that number is only going to grow. Imagine a world where the vast majority of the people are living their best lives, unencumbered by the debilitating conditions we've discussed in this book. This is my vision of the future that gives purpose to each day.

The Outer Limits of the Human Healthspan

Such thoughts lead to the question of how much is possible. That is, how far can we extend the human lifespan? And importantly, how much of that extra time will we be able to enjoy with sound minds and bodies? In other words, what are the outer limits of the human healthspan?

For those who seek answers to these questions, there is an entire industry devoted to longevity. This includes inquiries that are science based, as well as some theories that veer into science fiction with aspirations of one day becoming science fact. As you might imagine, NAD+ is quite the rage in both the hard science and pseudo-science circles of this community. I am often asked to speak at longevity conferences, and I'm always impressed with the passion of the attendees. But sometimes their passion overwhelms their reason, as when they suggest that humans will someday be able to live forever.

When I push back against this fantastical notion, they can be quite insistent, and I can get a little exasperated. "Okay, Bro. Agree to disagree?" I try to explain that nature is rather stubborn; throughout human history, 100 years has been an extreme outlier and 120 years seems to be the maximum Mother Nature allows. I don't believe we'll ever exceed that limit. Nor do I imagine we'd want to. However, I do believe we can make one century the norm for lifespan and that we can extend our healthspan, so those extra years will be worth living. But for that to happen, we'll need more than a generous supply of NAD+. We will need precision medicine.

Precision Medicine as the Key to Healthspan

By precision medicine, I mean precise diagnosis, precise targeting of the underlying causes of symptoms, and precise monitoring of progress. Conventional medicine is too imprecise, which is why treatment is so expensive and results are so apparently random. Medical treatment is also poorly executed in too many cases, which is why researchers from Johns Hopkins University[48] suggested in 2016 that medical errors

48 *https://www.npr.org/sections/health-shots/2016/05/03/476636183/death-certificates-under-count-toll-of-medical-errors*

might be the third leading cause of death in the United States. Yet, for some reason, patients tolerate vagaries in medical science, while they demand exactitude in less crucial aspects of life.

Take, for example, air travel. Imagine you were boarding a plane in Los Angeles, intending to arrive in New York five hours later. If the airline told you there was an 80 percent chance this outcome would result, but there was a 15 percent chance you'd land in Philadelphia and a five percent chance you'd wind up in Boston, would you take the flight? Of course not! You wouldn't even order a cup of coffee if you thought there was a five percent chance the barista would mess up your order. But patients accept medical treatment with huge caveats all the time.

Inaccuracies in medicine can have devastating consequences, especially for progressive diseases that get harder to treat over time. Were you aware that in the United States, five percent of all cancer patients, which comes to 86,500 individuals, are misdiagnosed every year? This means they receive the wrong treatments, if any, and suffer unnecessarily as their disease progresses, often to the death. If you have a loved one who's dealing with cancer, you cannot accept a five percent chance of a misdiagnosis.

Oncologists remind us that the earlier we catch cancer, the easier it is to treat and the greater the prognosis for recovery. But even if a doctor diagnoses your cancer in stage one, you've still got cancer. That's a full-blown, potentially fatal disease. We can be grateful we're not at stage three or four, but wouldn't it have been even better if the doctor had recognized systemic anomalies that might lead to cancer? Then, we'd be in a position to prevent cancer rather than treat it, so the prognosis would be even brighter.

But how do we make medicine more precise? As a microbiologist, I want to trace diseases back to their earliest origins. I don't want to wait until a disease is present in the tissues of an organ. I want to spot abnormalities when they first occur in the molecules of a patient's cells, so with a few proper adjustments, we can restore homeostasis and prevent disease. That is the purpose of biomarker testing, to which I have devoted many years of my career.

The Benefits of Biomarker Testing

Perhaps we should begin with the definition of a biomarker or biological marker. This is a measurable indicator of a biological state or condition. Scientists like me examine biomarkers found in blood, urine, or tissue samples to note whether molecular compounds are balanced or skewed in one direction of the other. Of course, in order to know whether a sample deviates from the norm, we have to have collected enough samples of heathy individuals to establish proper norms. One of the problems with contemporary medicine is that we usually take biomarkers from people who are complaining of poor health, so we run the risk of establishing abnormal norms.

As a data-driven scientist, I want to collect as many samples as possible from people in all stages of health, and index them according to those people's physical complaints. From this, we can start to see patterns emerging, as certain biomarkers will be shown to correspond consistently with certain conditions.

The relationship between certain biomarkers and unhealthy conditions has already been strongly established. For example, we know what biomarkers indicate oxidative stress, chronic inflammatory conditions, and cellular senescence (i.e., the cessation of cell division). A person's level of intracellular NAD+ is also an important biomarker for all the reasons we've discussed in this book: energy production, cellular respiration, cell division, cell signaling, and on and on.

At *Jinfiniti*, we have developed a panel of 20 essential biomarkers that are linked to age-related illnesses and metabolic dysfunctions. We urge anyone who wants to try *Vitality Boost* to test before taking the supplement. We understand that testing adds cost, but the extra expenditure delivers important benefits:

TESTING ESTABLISHES A BASELINE — When you are trying to become healthy, it's important to know your starting point. Just how low are your NAD+ levels? Perhaps your NAD+ is not deficient at all and some other condition is causing your symptoms. You'll also want to know what your other biomarkers indicate. It is highly unlikely that you would be suffering from low NAD+ and not have at least a few more skewed biomarkers. By identifying these, you can take a holistic approach to remedying your condition.

TESTING PINPOINTS AREAS OF TREATMENT — Would you rather use a shotgun or a laser? If you don't test, you can only have a vague idea of the causes for your condition and the possible remedies available. That forces you to take a shotgun approach, loading up on supplements that you might not need. This not only creates unnecessary expense, but it can cause confusion when you start to improve. What compounds actually caused the improvement? You can't really know, so you just keep loading up the shotgun, compounding your unnecessary expenses. (You'd have been better off to spring for the test in the beginning, which would have saved you money over time.) However, if you have clear biomarkers to target, you can be judicious about the remedies you choose.

TESTING ALLOWS YOU TO MEASURE YOUR PROGRESS — If you don't test and simply use the shotgun approach, you might still notice an improvement. But you won't know exactly where that improvement is coming from. You could also be fooled into thinking you're improving across the board, when in reality, a couple of stubborn conditions have persisted and will cause harm over time. On the other hand, if you test before supplementing, and test periodically afterwards, you can measure the changes in your biomarkers to ensure you are addressing the full scope of your issues.

It usually takes only two to four weeks for the supplements to raise your NAD. We advise another test at about the four-week mark. Once your NAD is optimized, you only need to test again two or three times a year. You may need to test with different regularity if your health status has significantly changed, or you have changed the types and dosage of NAD products, or other supplements, medicines, or lifestyle.

TESTING LETS YOU KNOW IF YOUR PRODUCTS ARE WORKING — This is a supremely important point. Not all supplements are the same. Different formulas and different delivery methods have different efficacy. I wish I could tell you how many times we've encountered someone who had trusted that NAD+ IVs or patches were the state-of-the-art delivery method, only to learn through testing that those techniques didn't raise their intracellular NAD+ levels. They thought they were buying the Mercedes Benz of NAD+ practices, but wound up with a used Saturn Ion. Imagine repeating an expensive and inconvenient process like an NAD+ IV time and again, accepting on faith that you were paying for the best possible method, then finding out you could have gotten far better results with our oral supplement, *Vitality Boost*.

TESTING HELPS YOU AVOID HARMFUL INTERVENTIONS — Here, we need to talk about medical interventions in general. NAD+ supplementation is incredibly safe, even when the methods are not optimal. But imagine that your doctor suspected a serious medical condition, but instead of testing for it, went with his gut and wrote you a prescription. If the doctor's gut is wrong, that prescription would do nothing to impede the progress of the disease while possibly causing harmful side effects. Or consider the doctor who only wants to treat the obvious symptoms but doesn't test for the underlying illness. Again, the disease progresses even though the symptoms might momentarily clear up.

TESTING CONTRIBUTES TO MEDICAL SCIENCE — As I alluded to above, the more medical data we have, the more we come to understand the norms for healthy homeostasis and the relationships between biomarkers and disease. By accumulating and analyzing data, we test the limits of our knowledge and make new discoveries which can be beneficial for patients in the future.

For these reasons and more, precision medicine is gaining traction in medical circles. But unfortunately, it's also become a buzzword bandied about by people who don't truly know what they are talking about and can't actually offer precise diagnostics.

Much of my earliest work was in oncology, where we were attempting to establish biomarkers for cancer. Thus, I started a precision medicine program more than 25 years ago. Today, *Jinfiniti* is the only company using precision medicine for NAD+ optimization and longevity programs. Others might talk about precision medicine, but they don't have the biomarker testing that *Jinfiniti* offers. Remember, I founded *Jinfiniti* as a biomarker testing company. We don't claim to be unique, but we offer the most comprehensive, advanced biomarker testing, as well as the most precise tracking for NAD+ optimization. I'm proud to be able to claim that *Jinfiniti* is the best one-stop shop for biomarker testing and NAD+ supplementation.

NAD+ Biomarkers Unlock the Key to Healthy Aging

Now, to return to the subject of healthspan. Think for a moment of all the manifestations of physical decline that we associate with aging. These conditions are bound to cross your mind:

- Chronic pain, such as sciatica, neuropathy, or joint pain
- Decreased energy
- Loss of mental sharpness
- Fatigue
- Muscle soreness
- Insulin resistance

Now, think of the diseases that come with old age. Your list is likely to include:

- Cardiovascular disease
- Adult-onset diabetes
- Arthritis
- Cancer
- Parkinson's disease
- Alzheimer's disease

What do all of these maladies have in common? They all have biomarkers, which we might refer to as the hallmarks of aging. These biomarkers inform us of the presence of inflammation, inefficient metabolism, low energy production on the cellular level, insufficient cell signaling, instability of genomes, oxidative stress, and other disfunctions. The one biomarker that consistently stands out as crucial to all these areas of decline is NAD+.

As we've discussed before, virtually every important cellular function requires NAD+. It's when we lose NAD+ that our functional decline on the cellular level begins. By restoring NAD+, we can reverse that functional decline. And since "functional decline" is simply a description of aging, it's natural to conclude that restoring NAD+ can reverse aging. To an extent.

We are not talking about *The Curious Case of Benjamin Button*, where a baby, born an old man, ages backwards until he's an infant. Naturally, there will be a limit to the degree that each individual will experience an "age reversal." But many of our clients report feeling 20 years younger or better. (That has been my personal experience.) And since the science behind NAD+ optimization is also young, we don't know how hard a stop we can put on aging. What happens when a 60-year-old resets his internal clock at 40 and begins to age at a slower pace? How much slower will he age and for how long will the rate of his aging be slower than normal? Perhaps the results will be like a science fiction story, where passengers in a faster-than-light spaceship age more slowly than the people on Earth. Movie fans might remember the 2014 science fiction film *Interstellar*. In one scene, space travelers who go down to the surface of a planet age more slowly than their crewmate who remains in orbit. They return to their ship after a few minutes to find their crewmate has become an elderly man. That's a little bit how I felt seeing my old classmates after I had taken *Vitality Boost* for more than a year. (But please, don't tell them!)

It's amusing to speculate, but at this point, all we have is speculation. It will take many years to collect the data necessary to understand how profoundly NAD+ optimization can impact human aging. But while we wait on those results, we might as well feel as youthful as possible.

CHAPTER 10

THE SYNERGY OF NAD+ OPTIMIZATION AND LIFESTYLE CHOICES

The New Eight Pillars

"It takes a tiny bit of willingness to follow this path, but many things distract us. This path is broad and steady, but we are conditioned to follow our thoughts down the countless sidetracks."

—Lao-Tzu, *Tao Te Ching*

Finally, we knew we had an effective supplement, and we could optimize levels of NAD+ in individuals of various ages in different states of health. We also knew that optimized NAD contributes to a strong healthspan. But our supplement is not a magic potion. It cannot correct for other factors that might undermine a person's health. In this way, NAD supplementation is essential but not sufficient. People suffering from a systemic imbalance that impedes their health and could potentially lead to disease must seek balance in their lives. Because we believe that NAD+ optimization works synergistically with other components of a healthy lifestyle, we urge our clients to modify their lifestyles in a way that sustains the healthspan that optimized NAD offers.

After giving this matter much thought, it occurred to me that we needed a new *Tao*, or Way, which we would call the *Tao of NAD*. The word *Tao* also lent itself to a clever acronym for the important stages of our process, as follows:

- **TEST** — Before you can go anywhere, you have to know where you are. As we mention in the previous chapter, precision testing of biomarkers is vitally important for understanding what you need to do to improve your health. You cannot be like our doctor friend who pumped himself full of niacin, then had to live with terrible insomnia. Testing at different intervals helps you fine tune your program as you go along, so you can enhance the benefits and avoid uncomfortable side effects.
- **ACT** — You must take charge of your healthspan by making the appropriate lifestyle choices. You must develop a plan and implement it. You must maintain a disciplined approach, which can be difficult in the beginning, but becomes easier as you begin to enjoy the benefits.
- **OPTIMIZE** — We always want to live in that "sweet spot" where are NAD levels remain in the optimum range. Consistent supplementation and periodic testing can ensure optimization even as we age. But we also want other aspects of our life to be optimized. We want to get optimal exercise, optimal sleep, and consume an optimal diet. We want to live, laugh, and love, all of which is easier when we stay on the path of the *Tao*.

This new path towards a maximized healthspan might also have Eight Pillars, that is, eight concepts for maintaining the benefits of NAD optimization. Though I am no Lao Tzu, here is my humble attempt at prescribing practices to optimize your optimization. You will note there is considerable overlap; that is the nature of synergy! These Eight Pillars, all capital Ps, will uphold your efforts to reap the benefits of an extended healthspan:

PREDICTIVE — If you are at risk of disease, don't you want to know? Especially if that knowledge could help you avert disaster? I've said before that I am data driven. I collect biometric data like one of those hoarders you see on reality TV, except that I don't leave it in a storage locker collecting dust. I analyze biomarkers, cross-referencing every possible combination to understand how they work individually and in tandem. Taken together, your biomarkers predict whether you will develop age-related illnesses. But they also provide a roadmap to optimal healthspan. To get where you're going, you must first know where you are! So, take the plunge and have a blood panel done. Then, follow up every so often, so you understand where you have progressed.

PROACTIVE — It's your healthspan, so you must take control! Educate yourself about NAD. Don't just take my word for it but look at other reputable studies. Then compare what the results say to your own experience of your energy, stamina, mood, mental clarity, and other important aspects of your health. Remember what we said about the panels: you are only as strong as your weakest link. Study your panels, learn what you must do to correct your deficiencies, and plan a course of action to strengthen areas of weakness.

PREVENTATIVE — Biomarkers are the keys to the prevention and treatment of countless ailments. But biomarkers don't tell the whole story. Your lifestyle choices can help you avoid diseases. So, if there is a biomarker you can tie to a poor diet or a sedentary lifestyle, to smoking or occupational stress, you now have vital information you can act upon. Modify your lifestyle and see what happens to that biomarker. Additionally, a biomarker might indicate the presence of subclinical disease, giving you the opportunity for early treatment, which is generally less expensive and more likely to produce a favorable outcome.

PRECISE — Generalized symptoms are the bane of any healthcare provider. If you go into a doctor and say you're feeling rundown, listless, and a bit spacy, how is that doctor likely to respond? Your description or your symptoms does not provide enough hard data to arrive at a diagnosis and formulate a treatment plan. This is where biomarkers come in. Biomarker data pinpoints deficiencies that impact systems. They tell a physician where and how the patient should be treated. Biomarkers improve the efficacy of treatment and avoid side effects from off-target recommendations. With precise biomarkers, there's no more shooting in the dark with the choice of a molecule or its dosing!

PERSONALIZED — One of the great complaints of patients is that the healthcare system is too impersonal. Patients often feel they're being force-fed generic remedies in a one-size-fits-all manner, instead of getting a solution tailored to their specific concerns. How health and longevity depend on solutions that suit an individual's genetics, lifestyle, and personality. Since NAD is foundational, it can help all other supplements work better, reducing the number of supplements taken and their cost. (Use a case study of someone who doesn't want to take a hundred pills a day. Dr. She can tell stories of clients who were able to cut down on the number of products used.)

PARALLEL — Holistic health depends on action along parallel tracks, all leading to an optimal healthspan. Therefore, you need programs for your diet, exercise, lifestyle modification, and NAD supplementation. A healthspan, like a chain, is only as strong as its weakest link. You need to attend to related issues simultaneously to create a synergistic effect that is not just an incremental improvement, but truly transformative.

PRIORITIZED — Taking a holistic approach does not mean treating all issues equally. We must prioritize the areas of our greatest deficiency to achieve the quickest possible turnaround in our health. This is an area where biomarker data are most useful. An in-depth panel, such as *Jinfiniti* provides before you start your NAD optimization, pinpoints the trouble spots, enabling you to properly target broader health issues. Symptoms of poor health have numerous causes, so if we're just operating off a vague understanding of symptoms, we could implement strategies that are slightly off-base. Like the proverbial dog who barks up the wrong tree, we don't realize that our prize is hiding elsewhere. Biomarkers, by themselves or in combination, tell a specific story and beg us for a targeted remedy.

PERSISTENT — Optimization is not a one-shot deal; it's a lifestyle. Imagine buying a new car, which runs great, then doing nothing to maintain it. If you never change the oil, refill your fluids, or adjust your tire pressure, how long will your car remain at peak performance? When it comes to cars, most of us understand that regular maintenance is necessary to get the longest possible life from our vehicle. We need to apply the same principles to our healthspan. It is not enough to optimize once and then let our body gather rust. Optimum health depends on consistent application of principles over the long haul. We also have to be resilient whenever we face disappointment. Life has a way of interrupting our best laid plans, so we can expect disruptions to our diet, exercise routines, and our quiet time. But we cannot let these disruptions overthrow our planning, so that chaos becomes the norm, and our performance goals seem distant and unattainable. When we slip or trip, we must pick ourselves back up again and recommit to our personalized program of holistic health. We must return to our uncarved block.

CHAPTER 11

CONCLUSION

"It is the ability of a tree to bend in the wind that keeps it from toppling. Our natural tenderness is our true strength."

—Lao-Tzu, *Tao Te Ching*

In my Preface, I mentioned how this book should be taken as a sort of guide to becoming more fully and deeply human. This is the ultimate promise of NAD+ optimization. By unlocking the full potential of our cellular processes, we can have more abundant energy and mental clarity. We can free ourselves from unnecessary suffering. We can live and love more passionately, pursuing our hopes and dreams. And, as the quotation from Lao-Tzu suggests, we can better deal with any tempests that life throws at us. We will not have to harden ourselves against the elements, but even under adversity, we can maintain the tenderness that makes us truly human.

Thus, there is little more to say than, "Good luck on your journey of a thousand miles." It has been my honor to point out the trailhead, but only you can walk the path. Your trail may wind, and you may face switchbacks as you climb, so it appears that you are making no progress. But eventually, you can attain a summit unique to you. From there, you can survey all that you've accomplished, and all that the world has placed at your feet. And you can take satisfaction in knowing you did it yourself.

FREQUENTLY ASKED QUESTIONS

For quick reference and basic understanding of common issues, I present this brief list of Frequently Asked Questions about NAD. I hope you'll find this useful as you implement the 8 Pillars of TAO into your healthspan extension plan. For a further understanding of *Jinfiniti*'s supplement formulations and biomarker tests, as well as science and blog items related to NAD, please visit www.jinfiniti.com or contact the company via email at: **hello@jinfiniti.com**.

What is NAD?

NAD is found in all living cells, from single-cell organisms to complex, multicellular systems like those in primates. It helps convert food to energy. It plays a crucial role in maintaining DNA integrity, helping repair damages to prevent cancer. It helps regulate our body's sleep/wake cycle through its

effect on circadian rhythm. Our cells' ability to create energy depend upon it. It transports electrons from molecule to molecule within the cells. NAD is what I call a "Foundational Supplement." Without it, other supplements and nutrients cannot do their work and we would quickly stop functioning as human beings.

NAD stands for nicotinamide adenine dinucleotide. It is a co-enzyme, and, as mentioned above, is found in all living cells. Along with the functions already cited, it also helps get rid of aging (senescent) cells, improves mitochondrial function, and supports the reduction of inflammation and free radicals. NAD catalyzes reactions for more than 500 enzymes, including those involved in the production of cellular energy (ATP). Deficient NAD levels are linked to a loss of function, vitality, and increased the risk of developing age-related diseases. Different terms are used for NAD. NAD+ is the oxidized form of NAD. When NAD+ is reduced, it becomes NADH, which carries electrons to the electron transport chain to generate ATP, the energy currency of the cell. Both NADH and NAD+ are important for optimal cellular function, but NAD+ is the more active form that participates in many biochemical reactions.

NAD was initially discovered in 1906, but it has seen an uptick in research that continues to show its importance in cell function and health benefits. Dr. Jin-Xiong She, Founder and Chief Scientific Officer of *Jinfiniti* Precision Medicine, left a prestigious career as an academic professor and eminent scientist to focus his talents exclusively on the study and development of ways to better understand and optimize this abundant and crucial molecule. Once he fully understood that without enough of this linchpin molecule we would be on the fast track to disease and death, he knew that his mission to help people extend their healthspan needed to center around NAD. To further our understanding and better address the body's need for NAD, he developed the world's first clinical test for NAD.

What Are the Signs of Low NAD?

The most common signs of deficient NAD include chronic fatigue, lack of energy, poor performance, lack of mental clarity, sleeping issues, and poor health in general. However, you may not show any symptoms while your NAD levels are already low.

What is the Best Way to Optimize NAD Levels?

The most efficient way is through oral supplementation with NAD precursors - building blocks that our cells use to make the NAD molecule.

The main NAD precursors on the market include nicotinamide mononucleotide (NMN) and nicotinamide riboside (NR). *Jinfiniti* data indicate that NMN works a little better than NR. However, *Jinfiniti*'s patented Vitality NAD+ Booster (with NMN, Creatine monohydrate, D- ribose and nicotinamide/ niacinamide) is by far more potent than both pure NMN and NR, not only for elevating NAD levels but more importantly for providing various health benefits.

Does Nicotinamide (NAM) Increase NAD?

Nicotinamide (NAM) is also called niacinamide, and some people may wrongfully call it niacin. NAM is a very inefficient NAD precursor. Clinical trials have shown that NAM can modestly increase NAD levels in about 30% of the individuals. Therefore, NAM is a poor NAD precursor. Furthermore, two terminal metabolites of nicotinamide (2PY and 4PY) have been shown to increase vascular inflammation and potentially cardiovascular risk. Therefore, taking high doses of nicotinamide with the hope to increase NAD levels is a poor choice.

Is Niacin a Good or Bad NAD+ Precursor?

Nicotinic acid (NA), commonly called niacin, is a compound that can be converted into NAD+. Niacin is a supplement and commonly prescribed drug to lower LDL cholesterol levels. It is well known that niacin is very effective in reducing LDL but its cardiovascular benefit is controversial.

Surprisingly, data from *Jinfiniti* showed that high dose niacin can increase NAD to levels that are much above the higher end of the optimal range and are bad for health. Very high levels of NAD associated with niacin use can increase vascular inflammation and risk for cardiovascular disease and may be responsible for insomnia. Niacin is not an ideal NAD+ precursor.

All niacin users should measure their NAD levels to find out whether their NAD levels are too high to decide whether they should reduce the dosage or to stop it completely.

Can I Use Any NAD Supplements From Any Vendor?

There are many different products, brands, and delivery routes. The products on the market are extremely variable in terms of efficacy, much of which has not been tested in clinical studies. Furthermore, a product that works well for one person may not work for others. You should find out whether your chosen product works for you by testing your NAD levels.

How Often Should I Test My NAD Levels?

It usually takes only 2-4 weeks to raise your NAD to the peak level. It's ideal to take a NAD test before starting a NAD optimization program. Then, to make sure that your chosen product is working, we advise another test 2-4 weeks after supplementation daily. Once your NAD is optimized, you only need to test again once every 6 months or so. You need to test more regularly if your health status has significantly changed, or you have changed the types and dosage of NAD products.

Is NAD Testing Needed for Everyone?

Yes. All adults are advised to take a NAD test to determine whether their NAD level is within the optimum range or if supplementation is needed. If you already take NAD supplements or other products, a test will determine whether or not they are working for you, and help you decide if you should change the product or dosage for better NAD optimization. This is essential because most NAD products on the market do not work as intended or cannot optimize NAD levels in most individuals. Children with health issues can also benefit from NAD testing and potentially supplementation.

Does IV Infusion of NAD+ Increase NAD Levels?

This is a complicated question. Yes, intravenous infusion of NAD+ can rapidly NAD+ levels in the plasma. However, it is rapidly degraded and there is almost nothing left after one since the half life of NAD+ in plasma is only six hours.

No, NAD+ IV does not increase intracellular NAD+ levels. *Jinfiniti*'s clinical studies and data from consumers unambiguously demonstrate that intravenous infusion of NAD+ does not increase NAD levels at all. There are potentially multiple reasons for this observation. First, the amount of infused NAD+ and the frequencies of infusion do not provide sufficient NAD+. Second, NAD+ is rapidly (within hours) degraded in the blood stream. Third, the NAD+ molecule is too big to get inside the cells. Therefore, NAD+ infusion is not the right choice for most consumers who wish to increase energy, performance, or longevity extension due to the high cost, lack of efficacy and potential side effects including rapid increase of C-reactive protein (CRP) after infusion in some 70% of customers.

However, IV infusion of NAD+ could be an useful treatment for certain health conditions and diseases including some neurological and infectious diseases. Individuals who receive IV NAD+ infusion should consider NAD testing and supplementation with oral precursors in addition to IV infusion.

Does Subcutaneous Injection of NAD+ Elevate NAD Levels?

Subcutaneous (SubQ) injection of NAD+ can modestly elevate NAD levels but rarely increase it to the optimum levels for maximum benefits. The efficacy certainly depends on the dosage and frequency of injection. It is advised that SubQ users of NAD+ check their NAD levels to determine whether their protocol is working for them. Due to the high cost, invasive nature of injections, and insufficient efficacy for SubQ NAD+.

Are There Health Risks or Side Effects to Taking NAD Supplements?

Side effects associated with taking safe dosages of high-quality NAD supplements are extremely rare. Minor stomach upset and skin rush are some side effects reported by a few individuals.

At What Age Do NAD Levels Begin to Decline?

Approximately 75% of teenagers have NAD levels above 40μM, the lower end of the optimum range, while 25% of the teenagers are already suboptimal or deficient in NAD. A sharp decline in NAD levels happens around 30 years of age in most people. Approximately 75% of individuals around 30 years are suboptimal or deficient in NAD. The decline continues as we age.

At What Age Should One Begin Taking NAD Supplements?

People of any age including very young children can take high quality and safe NAD supplements such as *Jinfiniti*'s Vitality NAD+ Booster. All adults after their 30s can and should supplement for NAD. It is ideal to take an NAD test before supplementation but it is absolutely essential to test NAD levels after any NAD treatment to determine whether the product is working for you and make some adjustment if necessary. For individuals younger than 20 years of age, testing for NAD levels is recommended before taking a supplement.

Does NAD Supplementation Interfere With My Regular Vitamin Regimen?

Since NAD and its precursors such as NMN and NR already exist in the body, it is very safe to take high quality NAD supplements. There is no known interference between NMN and other supplements. However, optimized NAD may improve the efficacy of other supplements or health optimization protocols.

Will I Feel a Difference After Taking NAD Supplements?

Yes, most people should notice some health benefits if their NAD level is optimized, meaning that their NAD levels are between 40µM and 100 µM. Those who get the most benefits usually have NAD levels between 50µM and 80µM. The most common benefits include improved energy, vitality, sleep, mental clarity/brain fog, joint health, insulin sensitivity, alcohol tolerance, sexual function, endurance and recovery as well as reduction in LDL, liver enzymes, inflammation, allergies and asthma, neurological conditions, autism symptoms, addiction, pain and aches, arthritis and many others. If you do not experience any health benefits after taking NAD therapies, it is highly likely that your NAD level is not in the optimum range or you are taking the wrong NAD product for you.

We recommend that you try *Jinfiniti*'s Vitality NAD+ Booster formula and get your NAD level tested using the Intracellular NAD test or the AgingSOS advanced panel test. *Jinfiniti* can work with you to find a personalized solution.

What are Zombie Cells and Can NAD Help?

Senescence is a biological process in which cells stop dividing and enter a state of permanent growth arrest. This is a natural process that occurs as we age and is thought to be a protective mechanism that helps prevent the development of cancer. However, as we get older, the accumulation of senescent cells can contribute to a variety of age-related diseases, such as cardiovascular disease, osteoporosis, neurodegenerative diseases and cancer. Senescent cells, also called "Zombie" cells by biohackers, are cells that have entered a state of senescence but have not been cleared by the body. These cells can accumulate in tissues and organs and secrete harmful substances, known as senescence-associated phenotype (SASP), which contribute to chronic inflammation and tissue damage. This can lead to a variety of age-related diseases and can accelerate the aging process.

Of interest to the NAD topic is the link between NAD and senescence. NAD plays a very important role in the regulation of cell proliferation, cell cycle arrest and the secretion of SASP by senescence. Therefore, optimization of NAD levels can help reduce senescent cells and SASP secretion.

Can Cancer Patients or Survivors Increase Their NAD Levels Safely?

The relationship between NAD and cancer is complex and multifaceted, reflecting the intricate nature of cancer biology and the diversity of cancer types. On one hand, NAD can potentially increase proliferation of cells including cancer cells. On the other hand, NAD has the potential to actually benefit cancer patients through at least four mechanisms:

1. NAD has been shown to be essential to the killing of cancer cells by antitumor CD8 T cells.
2. Increased tumor cell growth may turn a cold tumor into a hot tumor that responds better to chemotherapy and is associated with better survival.
3. NAD is known to reduce inflammation which has a negative impact on patient treatment outcome.
4. NAD can increase the overall health and vitality of cancer patients so that they can fight cancer better. The overall impact of NAD on patients with active cancer certainly depends on the condition of the patients and the treatment protocols

To learn more about NAD and cancer, you can read a comprehensive blog here: NAD and Cancer: NAD and Cancer: ***NAD and Cancer: What We Know and What We Don't - Jinfiniti Precision Medicine***

It is also important to point out that NAD does not cause cancer and in contrary optimized NAD levels can help cancer prevention by improving repair of damaged DNA that is the major underlying risk for all types of cancer.

Please visit www.jinfiniti.com for the most updated information and topics that are not covered in this FAQ.

ABOUT THE AUTHOR

Dr. Jin-Xiong She is a world-renowned scientist, entrepreneur, and visionary in the fields of aging, longevity, and precision medicine. With a distinguished career spanning over four decades, Dr. She has revolutionized our understanding of human biomarkers, genomic medicine, and healthspan optimization.

Born and educated in China, he earned his PhD in France before launching a successful academic career in the United States. At the University of Florida, he rose to the rank of Endowed Professor, Division Chief of Experimental Pathology, and Director of Research at the Diabetes Center. Later, as a Georgia Research Alliance Eminent Scholar, he founded the Center for Biotechnology and Genomic Medicine, one of the world's first institutions dedicated to genomic medicine.

A prolific scientist, Dr. She has authored over 400 peer-reviewed papers, amassed more than 20,000 citations, and secured over $100 million in research funding. Now, as the founder and CEO of *Jinfiniti* Precision Medicine, he pioneers biomarker-driven solutions to extend healthspan, proving that aging is not a destiny but a choice. He is a sought-after keynote speaker, a featured expert in the documentary Biohack Yourself, and the host of the Healthspan Insider Podcast, where he shares cutting-edge insights on longevity and biohacking.

He is eager to point out that *Jinfiniti* is not a company just selling supplements and tests. "We teach a lifestyle and a philosophy. That's why it was important to me to write this book."

When he's not pushing the boundaries of human health, Dr. She enjoys gardening, raising chickens, and playing highly competitive tennis—fueled, of course, by his own health optimization strategies. "My goal is to be serving aces at 100," he says. And if his research is any indication, he's well on his way.

Dr. She lives in Augusta, Georgia, with his wife, Boying, and their two daughters, Lily and Jasmine.

www.ingramcontent.com/pod-product-compliance
Lightning Source LLC
Chambersburg PA
CBHW022052020426
42335CB00012B/661

9781965971161